Rapid
Neurology and
Neurosurgery

Rapid Neurology and Neurosurgery

Kumar Abhinav

BSc (Hons.), MBBS, MRCS (Eng)
Specialty Registrar
Department of Neurosurgery
Frenchay Hospital
Bristol, UK

Richard Edwards

BSc (Hons.), MBBS, FRCS (Neuro.Surg), MD
Consultant Neurosurgeon
& Senior Clinical Lecturer (University of Bristol)
Department of Neurosurgery
Frenchay Hospital
Bristol, UK

Alan Whone

MBChB, MRCP, PhD
Senior Lecturer (University of Bristol) & Consultant Neurologist
Department of Neurology
Frenchay Hospital
Bristol, UK

⊛WILEY-BLACKWELL

A John Wiley & Sons, Ltd., Publication

This edition first published 2012 © 2012 by John Wiley & Sons, Ltd

Wiley-Blackwell is an imprint of John Wiley & Sons, formed by the merger of Wiley's global Scientific, Technical and Medical business with Blackwell Publishing.

Registered office: John Wiley & Sons, Ltd, The Atrium, Southern Gate, Chichester, West Sussex, PO19 8SQ, UK

Editorial offices: 9600 Garsington Road, Oxford, OX4 2DQ, UK
                       The Atrium, Southern Gate, Chichester, West Sussex, PO19 8SQ, UK
                       111 River Street, Hoboken, NJ 07030-5774, USA

For details of our global editorial offices, for customer services and for information about how to apply for permission to reuse the copyright material in this book please see our website at www.wiley.com/wiley-blackwell.

The right of the author to be identified as the author of this work has been asserted in accordance with the UK Copyright, Designs and Patents Act 1988.

Library of Congress Cataloging-in-Publication Data

Abhinav, Kumar.
Rapid neurology and neurosurgery / Kumar Abhinav, Richard Edwards, Alan Whone.
      p. ; cm. – (Rapid series)
   Includes bibliographical references and index.
      ISBN 978-0-470-65443-9 (pbk. :alk. paper)
      I. Edwards, Richard (Richard John) II. Whone, Alan. III. Title. IV. Series: Rapid series.
      [DNLM: 1.   Nervous System Diseases–Handbooks. 2.   Neurosurgical Procedures–Handbooks.
3.   Trauma, Nervous System–Handbooks. WL 39]

   616.80076–dc23

                                                                    2012009836

A catalogue record for this book is available from the British Library.

Wiley also publishes its books in a variety of electronic formats. Some content that appears in print may not be available in electronic books.

Cover image: iStock © Sebastian Kaulitzki
Cover design by Fortiori Design

Set in 7.5/9.5pt Frutiger-Light by Thomson Digital, Noida, India
Printed and bound in Malaysia by Vivar Printing Sdn Bhd

1   2012

Contents

List of Abbreviations, vii

Preface, xi

Acknowledgements, xiii

PART I The basics
1   About this book and how to use it, 3
2   Basic neuroanatomy, 4
3   Neurological history, examination, signs and localisation, 7
4   Neurological investigations, 21

PART II Complaints: Face-to-face with the patient
5   Headache, 31
6   Blackouts, 34
7   Visual disturbances, 36
8   Dizziness and vertigo, 39
9   Weak legs, 41
10   Numbness and sensory disturbance, 44
11   Gait assessment and disturbance, 46

PART III Conditions: Applying the basics
12   Headache, 51
13   Transient ischaemic attacks (TIAs), 55
14   Stroke I: Thromboembolic stroke and syndromes, 59
15   Stroke II: Intracerebral haemorrhage, 65
16   Stroke III: Subarachnoid haemorrhage, 68
17   Epilepsy, 75
18   Multiple sclerosis, 80
19   Parkinson's disease and other related syndromes, 84
20   Other movement disorders, 88
21   Central nervous system infections: Meningitis, 91
22   Central nervous system infections: Cerebral abscess, 94
23   Radiculopathy and disc herniation, 97
24   Peripheral neuropathies' syndromes, 100
25   Common peripheral nerve lesions: Mononeuropathies, 104
26   Motor neurone disease (MND), 108
27   Myasthenia gravis and Lambert–Eaton myasthenic syndrome, 111
28   Diseases of the muscle, 114
29   Alzheimer's disease and other dementia syndromes, 118
30   Raised intracranial pressure and herniation syndromes, 122
31   Coma and brainstem death, 127

32   Head injury: General approach and management, 130

33   Head injury: Subdural haematoma, skull fractures and contusions, 135

34   Head injury: Extradural haematoma, 141

35   Spinal injuries and spinal cord syndromes, 144

36   CNS neoplasia, 151

37   Hydrocephalus, 155

Appendices

Appendix 1   Management of status epilepticus (SE), 163

Appendix 2   Glasgow Coma Scale (GCS), 164

Appendix 3   Primary neuroepithelial tumours of the central nervous system, 166

Appendix 4   Other tumours affecting the central nervous system, 173

Index, 181

List of Abbreviations

ABC	Airways and breathing and circulation
AD	Alzheimer's disease
ADEM	Acute disseminated encephalomyelitis
ADHD	Attention deficit hyperactivity disorder
AED	Antiepileptic drug
AF	Atrial fibrillation
ALS	Amyotrophic lateral sclerosis
APP	Amyloid precursor protein
ASDH	Acute subdural haematoma
AVMs	Arteriovenous malformations
BNF	British National Formulary
BPV	Benign positional vertigo
CAA	Cerebral amyloid angiopathy
CADASIL	Cerebral autosomal dominant arteriopathy with subcortical infarcts and leukoencephalopathy
CBF	Cerebral blood flow
CES	Cauda equina syndrome
CIDP	Chronic inflammatory demyelinating polyneuropathy
CMAP	Compound muscle action potential
CN	Cranial nerve
CNS	Central nervous system
CPP	Cerebral perfusion pressure
CSDH	Chronic subdural haematoma
CT	Computed tomography
CTA	CT angiography
CTS	Carpal tunnel syndrome
CVR	Cerebral vascular resistance
DAI	Diffuse axonal injury
DBS	Deep brain stimulation
DIND	Delayed ischaemic neurological deficit
DVLA	Driver and Vehicle Licensing Agency
DVT	Deep venous thrombosis
EEG	Electroencephalogram
EMG	Electromyography
EMQ	Extended matching questions
ET	Essential tremor
ETV	Endoscopic third ventriculostomy
EVD	External ventricular drain
FTD	Frontotemporal dementia

FVC	Forced vital capacity
GCA	Giant cell arteritis
GBM	Glioblastoma multiforme
GBS	Guillian–Barré syndrome
GCS	Glasgow Coma Scale
GTC	Generalised tonic–clonic
HACE	High altitude cerebral oedema
ICH	Intracerebral haemorrhage
ICP	Intracranial pressure
IIH	Idiopathic intracranial hypertension
INO	Internuclear opthalmoplegia
IVIG	Intravenous immunoglobulin
LACS	Lacunar stroke
LEMS	Lambert–Eaton myasthenic syndrome
LBD	Lewy body dementia
LMN	Lower motor neurone
LOC	Loss of consciousness
LP	Lumbar puncture
LP	Lumboperitoneal
MAP	Mean arterial pressure
MCI	Mild cognitive impairment
MCQ	Multiple choice questions
MDT	Multidisciplinary team
MG	Myasthenia gravis
MND	Motor neurone disease
MRA	MR angiography
MRC	Medical Research Council
MRI	Magnetic Resonance Imaging
MS	Multiple sclerosis
MUPs	Motor unit potentials
NAHI	Non-accidental head injury
NCS	Nerve conduction studies
NMJ	Neuromuscular junction
NPH	Normal pressure hydrocephalus
OCSP	Oxford Community Stroke Project
OSCE	Objective Structured Clinical Examinations
PACS	Partial anterior circulation stroke
PBP	Progressive bulbar palsy
PCC	Prothrombin complex concentrate
PD	Parkinson's disease
PE	Pulmonary embolism
PEG	Percutaneous endoscopic gastrostomy

PFO	Patent foramen ovale
PLS	Primary lateral sclerosis
PMA	Progressive muscular atrophy
PNS	Peripheral nervous system
POCS	Posterior circulation stroke
PPMS	Primary progressive multiple sclerosis
PRES	Posterior reversible encephalopathy syndrome
PTA	Posttraumatic amnesia
RAPD	Relative afferent pupillary defect
RAS	Reticular activating system
REZ	Root entry zone
RRMS	Relapsing/remitting multiple sclerosis
RTA	Road traffic accidents
SACD	Subacute combined degeneration of the cord
SAH	Subarachnoid haemorrhage
SCI	Spinal cord injury
SCM	Sternocleidomastoid
SE	Status epilepticus
SEM	Spinal extradural metastases
SPMS	Secondary progressive multiple sclerosis
TACS	Total anterior circulation stroke
TBI	Traumatic brain injury
TIAs	Transient ischaemic attacks
TN	Trigeminal neuralgia
UMN	Upper motor neurone
VA	Ventriculoatrial
VP	Ventriculoperitoneal

Preface

My late grandfather, a university professor, used to talk about the so-called 'ideal' students, who read extensively on a topic prior to attending the relevant lecture, made their own 'notes' in their own 'words' in a summarised fashion, which they subsequently memorised in the lead up to the exams. This inspirational philosophy with respect to teaching and the 'ideal' learning method can be difficult to adhere to as a modern medical student, where the ever-increasing breadth of the curriculum makes it difficult to both identify the pertinent information and then assimilate it in preparation for the exams.

Our objective was to put together a book in a condensed format, which gave the necessary basic information for building a solid foundation in neurology and neurosurgery required by medical students and junior doctors, and then followed it up with sections on presenting complaints and all the key clinical conditions. This book aims to simplify information in specialties traditionally considered 'difficult', to which medical students have variable and usually limited exposure, and to facilitate focused exam preparation. We really hope differential diagnoses tables, a consistent feature across this book, are helpful particularly for OSCE and EMQ sections of the exam and are used to refresh knowledge from other cross-referenced chapters during revision.

We sincerely hope this easy-to-use and concise book with ample practical information is useful for exams and as a reference guide on the wards and clinics for medical students, junior doctors and other health professionals in neurology and neurosurgery.

Kumar Abhinav
Richard Edwards
Alan Whone

Acknowledgements

We are indebted to all those who provided helpful advice at different stages of the production of the book. We are also grateful to the medical students and junior doctors who provided invaluable advice regarding improving the contents of the book. Specifically, we would like to acknowledge the following at Frenchay Hospital, Bristol: Mr Kristian Aquilina, Consultant Neurosurgeon for authoring the chapters on meningitis and cerebral abscess; Dr Philip Clatworthy, Specialist registrar in Neurology and Stroke Medicine, for his contribution towards the chapters on transient ischaemic attacks and thromboembolic stroke and syndromes, and Mr Devindra Ramnarine, Senior registrar in Neurosurgery, for his feedback regarding the chapter on radiculopathy and disc herniation. We would further like to thank all our colleagues at the Wiley-Blackwell: in particular, Martin Davies for his support through the initial stages of the book proposal and Laura Murphy for her guidance through the preparation of the manuscript. Finally, we are immensely thankful to our partners and families for their encouragement and patience through the preparation of the book and particularly to Melanie Yoogalingam for her help and support throughout this endeavour.

Part I
The basics

1   About this book and how to use it

The principal purpose of this book is to act as a quick revision tool for medical students approaching finals or other undergraduate neurology/neurosurgery exams. Although the book is intended as a quick revision tool, using it diligently and devoting time to understanding the basic concepts outlined herein will allow you to neurologically flourish rather than simply pass exams. The book is designed for both the newer type of written exams, including multiple choice questions (MCQ) as well as the extended matching questions (EMQ), and traditional exams requiring long and short answers. This book is also designed to prepare you for the Objective Structured Clinical Examinations (OSCE); in particular, Part II is geared towards this purpose.

The book is divided into three parts. Part I gives you the necessary basic principles and facts essential for building a foundation in clinical neurology/neurosurgery at an undergraduate level. Only clinically relevant neuroanatomy is presented along with an introduction to the topics of neurological history, examination and investigations. In particular, we have tried to simplify neuroradiological concepts and presented the rationale for using different imaging modalities.

Part II is very much geared towards the OSCE and the viva voce exams in finals. This section consists of chapters dealing with various presenting complaints. Lists of *focussed and discriminating* questions for determining the *important differential diagnoses* are included in these chapters along with tables listing the relevant disease entities in order of incidence. Please note, however, that you will also be expected to ask other relevant questions not listed in the chapters while taking a detailed history, including past medical history, drug history and social history. Additional important clinical information for each presenting complaint is included. The tables of potential differential diagnoses are supplemented by information on basic investigations and management. *Again, in an exam setting you will have to be guided by the clinical information and suggest a list of focussed and relevant investigations!* This part of the book can also act as a worthy quick reference on wards and in clinics.

Part III presents the important clinical neurological and neurosurgical conditions with focussed pertinent clinical information. Neurological topics are presented first followed by neurosurgical topics with the exception of the chapter on subarachnoid haemorrhage, which is included under 'stroke'. Part III like other parts is interspersed with sentences beginning with '*Remember . . .* ' and designed to highlight key facts from the chapter. At the end of each chapter there is a list of common differential diagnoses (up to a maximum of four–five) for the particular condition described. General clinical details are provided, including, where applicable, information that can be used to distinguish between or exclude the alternative conditions. This should be of particular help for the EMQ section of the exam and will also prove useful in the OSCE when presenting a list of potential differential diagnoses.

Some of the chapters in the book may not strictly follow the format as laid out above and will generally be due to the nature of the topic and thereby the limitations of presenting it in a specific format.

We hope that the format; organisation and simple language employed will facilitate quick and effective revision and will help you perform well in all sorts of undergraduate examinations. Moreover, we trust this book will permit a better understanding of the basic concepts underpinning neurology and neurosurgery and thus provide a firm basis upon which to build your clinical neurological/neurosurgical expertise as you journey through your medical career.

Good Luck!

2   Basic neuroanatomy

The following section aims to present only the very relevant anatomical information.

Cortical anatomy
Figure 2.1 demonstrates the following relevant key areas on the cortical surface:
- *Primary motor cortex*: Situated anterior to central sulcus (frontal lobe) in the precentral gyrus; involved in contralateral motor function—Brodmann's (Br.) Area 4.
- *Primary somatosensory cortex*: Situated posterior to central sulcus (parietal lobe) in the postcentral gyrus; involved in contralateral sensory function—Br. Areas 1, 2 and 3.
- *Motor speech area*: In the dominant hemisphere only (left hemisphere for right-handed subjects and usually left hemisphere for left-handed people); anatomically situated in the inferior frontal gyrus (pars triangularis and opercularis); also known as 'Broca's area' and involved in speech output—Br. Area 44.
- *Wernicke's area*: In the dominant hemisphere; anatomically situated in the supramarginal gyrus—Br. Area 40 (part of inferior parietal lobule) and posterior part of superior temporal gyrus; involved in comprehension of speech.
- *Primary visual cortex*: In the occipital lobe adjacent to the calcarine sulcus—Br. Area 17; part of the visual pathway.

> *Remember: The association between dominant hemisphere and speech areas and therefore a further important point about ascertaining handedness of patients at the beginning of obtaining a neurological history.*

Brainstem and cranial nerves (CN)
The midbrain is the most rostral part of the brainstem; CN III (oculomotor) and IV (trochlear) arise from the midbrain. The pons is situated between the midbrain and the medulla with CN V (trigeminal), VI (abducens), VII (facial) and VIII (vestibulocochlear) nerve entering into

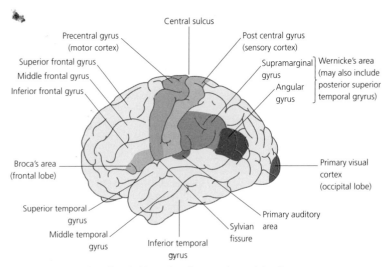

Figure 2.1 Lateral surface of cerebral hemisphere demonstrating cortical surface anatomy.

or exiting from ventral pons. The medulla is caudal to pons being continuous with spinal cord. Fibres of the CN IX (glossopharyngeal), X (vagus) and XII (hypoglossal) nerves enter into or exit from the ventral aspect of the medulla. The basic clinical features of lesions associated with cranial nerves are presented in Table 3.3.

> *Remember: An easier simplified way of remembering the site of entering or exiting of CN from brainstem is 2, 4 and 4, i.e. apart from first two cranial nerves, CN III and IV from midbrain with V–VIII from pons and IX–XII from medulla.*

Cerebellum

Cerebellum consists of the midline vermis, two cerebellar hemispheres and a flocculonodular lobe. Primary role of the cerebellum concerns the planning and fine-tuning of the movements. The cerebellum exercises its influence on the contralateral upper motor neurones in the cerebral cortex and brainstem. The vermis specifically has a role in trunk muscle control with lesions resulting in truncal ataxia.

> *Remember cerebellar lesions result in ipsilateral deficit.*

Vascular anatomy (cranial)

Figure 2.2 demonstrates the Circle of Willis at the base of the brain. CNS arterial supply is provided by a pair of internal carotid arteries (dividing into terminal branches of middle and anterior cerebral arteries) and a pair of vertebral arteries (uniting to form midline basilar artery at the junction between pons and medulla) forming the Circle of Willis. In terms of cerebral hemisphere, the blood supply is grossly as follows: anterior cerebral artery predominantly supplies the medial surface of the frontal and parietal lobes, including the motor

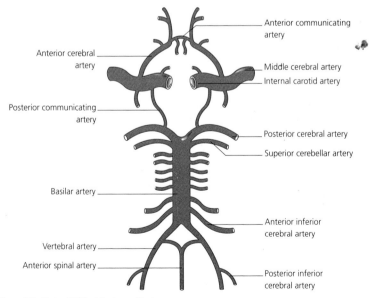

Figure 2.2 Circle of Willis at the base of brain.

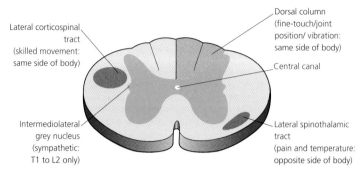

Figure 2.3 Cross section of spinal cord.

and sensory cortices for the contralateral lower limb; middle cerebral artery with the largest cortical territory supplies almost the whole of the lateral surface of frontal, parietal and temporal lobes, including the speech areas in the dominant lobe, primary motor and sensory cortices for the contralateral whole body excluding the lower limb; posterior cerebral artery (derived from basilar artery) supplies the inferomedial temporal lobe and the occipital lobe, including the visual cortex. The vertebrobasilar system as a whole supplies brainstem, cerebellum and occipital lobe.

With respect to internal capsule, the blood supply is derived from anterior choroidal artery arising from internal carotid artery, lateral striate branch of middle cerebral artery and recurrent artery of Heubner arising from anterior cerebral artery. The blood supply of basal ganglia is also derived from these arteries.

Spinal cord

The vascular supply of the spinal cord is derived from radicular arteries arriving from the aorta. Artery of Adamkiewicz is the main arterial supply for the spinal cord from T8 to conus. Midthoracic region being a watershed zone is susceptible to vascular injury leading to ischemia or infarct. Figure 2.3 demonstrates a cross section from the spinal cord, including the intermediolateral column, representing sympathetic outflow and present from T1–L2. It is worth reviewing briefly the anatomy of the three tracts as outlined below from a basic Neuroanatomy text. The basic clinical information regarding these three tracts is as below:

- *Lateral corticospinal tract*: Skilled movement (serving ipsilateral side).
- *Lateral spinothalamic tract*: Pain and temperature sensation (serving contralateral side).
- *Dorsal column*: Fine touch, joint position and vibration sense (serving ipsilateral side).

Peripheral nervous system

Important muscle groups with their spinal roots, named nerve supply and actions to test, are summarised in Table 3.5. Similarly, a dermatomal map demonstrating the dermatomes needing examination during a routine neurological exam is included in Chapter 3.

3   Neurological history, examination, signs and localisation

This chapter is not intended to be exhaustive but rather is a brief summary of taking a neurological/neurosurgical history and performing a neurological examination. Here, we provide an overview of the process and a framework which allows a neurological diagnosis to be reached.

One classical way of coming to a list of potential differential diagnoses when faced with a neurological/neurosurgical patient is to adopt the so-called *where, what* and *why* approach.

'Where'

It is often the case that the neurologist or neurosurgeon, when confronted with a patient, will first ask themselves, *where is the lesion?*, meaning where is the predominant focus of pathology within the neurological system.

The lesion may be at a single focus within the nervous system, such as entrapment of the median nerve at the wrist in the case of carpal tunnel syndrome or entrapment of an L5 nerve root in a patient with foot drop. Alternatively, the lesion may be multifocal, as in multiple sclerosis (MS) where demyelinating plaques may be found throughout the brain and spinal cord, or it may be diffuse or generalised, as in the case of encephalopathic patient with a reduced level of consciousness secondary to a systemic infection or metabolic derangement.

In some instances, gross localisation is very straightforward, for example, in a patient with traumatic brain injury post a road traffic accident, it is relatively implicit to focus localisation within the brain. In case of a patient complaining of weak legs (see Chapter 9), the problem could however variably be within the brain, brainstem, spinal cord (*central nervous system* (CNS)) or within the anterior horn cell, nerve root, lumbar sacral plexus, peripheral nerves or neuromuscular junction (*peripheral nervous system* (PNS)) or be isolated to skeletal muscle. In the latter scenario, the neurological examination is pivotal to localising the problem where, for example, upper motor neurone (UMN) signs will point to a problem in the central nervous system and lower motor neurone (LMN) signs will point to a problem in the peripheral nervous system. The distribution of signs will also point towards the potential site of the lesion; therefore, hemisphere lesions usually lead to *contralateral* weakness affecting face, arms and legs, variably depending on the exact site of the lesion, whereas a cord lesion usually produces *bilateral* weakness with possible evidence of LMN signs at the level of the lesion and UMN signs below the level of the lesion with a sensory level. Patients may present with typical syndromes (Table 3.1) observed with pathology in different parts of the CNS, thereby further helping in localisation (also refer to Chapter 35).

'What'

Having decided where the lesion lies, the next question to consider is *what is the problem?* Here we are thinking particularly of the aetiological group to which the potential diagnosis belongs. This is typically based upon the temporal sequence of events largely elicited by obtaining the history of the presenting complaint (Table 3.2).

'Why'

Having decided where the potential lesion lies and also to which causative group the diagnosis may belong, the next step is to consider *why might this disease or entity have occurred?*. For example, the patient presenting with acute onset of right arm weakness and language disturbance is likely to have an abnormality localising to the left frontal lobe with the sudden onset suggesting a vascular cause. The question then arises regarding the reason for the occurrence of the vascular event. With a preceding history of trauma, an extradural haemorrhage may be the explanation, whereas a past history of smoking, diabetes and hypertension might point more towards an ischaemic stroke. This gathering of

Table 3.1 Key areas within CNS with description of clinical syndromes related to pathology

Relevant areas within CNS	Clinical syndromes related to pathology
Frontal lobe	Dominant frontal lobe only (Broca's area): *Broca's* or *motor* or *expressive* or *non-fluent* dysphasia with intact comprehension of written and spoken language but reduced verbal output with difficulty in putting words together and difficulty with repetition
	Primary motor cortex: Contralateral hemiparesis or hemiplegia
	Premotor (anterior to primary motor cortex) and supplementary motor cortex: Apraxia (i.e. performance of movements is impaired despite normal strength) as this area plays a role in contralateral motor programming
	Prefrontal area: Frontal lobe syndrome (problems with behaviour and cognition; intelligence and memory; apathy, including lack of motivation and abulia, i.e. lack of initiative or awareness) usually resulting from a large unilateral or bilateral lesions
Parietal lobe	Primary somatosensory cortex: Problem with perceiving somatic sensation on contralateral side of body
	Superior parietal lobule (usually with *dominant hemisphere* lesions): Usually result in ideomotor apraxia (inability to carry out tasks on command despite absence of motor deficit or weakness) or constructional apraxia (inability to copy a diagram) or astereognosia (inability to recognise an object without looking at it, for example a coin in the palm of a patient with eyes closed)
	Inferior parietal lobule (angular and supramarginal gyrus) in *right hemisphere*: Contralateral neglect (asomatognosia) despite intact somatic sensation, i.e. patients neglect the left side of body including dressing or looking after it; classically these patients when asked to draw a clock face only draw numbers on the right side. With left parietal lobe lesion, contralateral neglect is uncommon
	Inferior parietal lobule *in left or dominant hemisphere*: Gerstmann's syndrome (finger agnosia, i.e. inability to recognise finger by name; agraphia without alexia, i.e. cannot write but can read; left–right disorientation and acalculia, i.e. inability to perform simple arithmetic calculations); with angular gyrus lesions (alexia, i.e. inability to read or comprehend written text and agraphia, i.e. inability to write); supramarginal gyrus and posterior part of superior temporal gyrus in dominant lobe (*Wernicke's or fluent or sensory or receptive aphasia* characterised by fluent speech without meaning)
Occipital lobe	Contralateral homonymous haemianopia with macular sparing results with lesions of primary visual cortex, usually due to occlusion of a branch of posterior cerebral artery (for field defects associated with other sites, see Chapter 7)
Cerebellum	Unilateral cerebellar hemisphere lesions: Ipsilateral gait ataxia (impaired heel to toe test and broad-based gait), problem with coordination (intention tremor on finger to nose, i.e. increase in tremor amplitude as target is approached; dysdiadochokinesia on repeated movements and impaired heel to shin test)
	Cerebellar vermis: Truncal ataxia

Refer to Chapter 2 and Figure 2.1 therein.

Table 3.2 Potential causative groupings along with brief temporal and other clues associated with a particular aetiological group

Aetiology	Characteristics/clues
Traumatic	Preceding history of trauma. Symptoms are typically acute but may, as in the case of chronic subdural haematoma, evolve over time
Vascular	Typically indicated by *abrupt* nature of onset, reaching maximum severity from outset
Infective	Typically a history evolving over days to weeks, although may evolve over months or be chronic. Supported by systemic markers of infection like raised white cell count or CRP/ESR
Metabolic	Typically symptoms evolve over days to weeks, although may be episodic or chronic
Malignant	Often symptoms evolve over weeks to months and may be due to direct tumour effects or as a paraneoplastic phenomena
Degenerative	Typically degenerative diseases evolve over months to years
Genetic	May be suggested by family history and typically symptoms evolve over months to years
Iatrogenic	This may be acute, subacute or chronic but clues are from the past medical history and history of medication exposure
Idiopathic	A causative category ascribed by a process of exclusion
Psychogenic	Be wary of ascribing a psychogenic cause, although very important to identify if this is the explanation

information regarding such associated factors should be covered in the history of the presenting complaint and other components such as the past medical history, the medication list, family history and social history.

The neurological history

Many of the questions pertinent to be asked when considering patient complaining of specific neurological symptoms are covered in Parts II and III of this book dealing with presenting complaints and specific disease entities, which may be referred to when confronted with specific neurological complaints. Below are some additional points that should be included in the medical student or junior doctor clerking when obtaining a neurological history.

In addition to detailing the patient's name, age, occupation and marital status, in a neurological history it is also common to record patient's handedness. Handedness suggests the dominant (language functioning) hemisphere of the brain, where nearly all right-handed people are left hemisphere dominant whereas only approximately 70% of left-handed people are left hemisphere dominant. Further understanding of patient's handedness will increase understanding of impairment the patient may be experiencing due to their deficit. For example, a patient with right body predominant Parkinson's disease who is right-handed will typically have greater impairment in fine finger function than a patient with left body predominant Parkinson's disease who is right-handed.

Complaint and history of the presenting complaint (see Part II)

Complaints may concern problems with senses, including sight, smell, hearing and taste. Other complaints may include blackouts, dizziness, headache, numbness, paraesthesia (pins and needles) and weakness in arms or legs. These are covered in detail in Part II. Disturbances with cognition, speech, swallowing and bowel or bladder function may also be reported. Psychiatric symptoms may also be present. A full history of presenting complaint is warranted, including mode of onset, provoking or triggering causes and progression of symptoms, for example gradual (with a slowly growing tumour) or rapid (e.g. in a vascular event like stroke). Also record the associated factors, for example in the case of a migraine headache, the associated factors of photophobia and nausea.

Past medical history
Events from the past medical history are often useful in understanding why patients may have developed a particular disease. Check regarding meningitis, foreign travel and previous history of CNS trauma (minor or major, for example with reference to extradural or subdural haematoma). Past medical history may also help localise the lesion and point to the causative aetiology, for example the patient with a recent history of tooth abscess and dental extraction in preceding weeks who then develops focal onset of seizures affecting the right hand may have a brain abscess affecting the left motor strip.

Medication history
Neurological symptoms as a side effect of medication are extremely common. A detailed list of the medications (including anticonvulsants, antidepressants or antipsychotics), the dose and frequency of administration, as well as documentation of previous medication exposures is extremely important, for example a patient presenting with numbness of both feet evolving over months who has had chemotherapy in the preceding year may have a peripheral sensory axonal neuropathy secondary to chemotherapy. Isoniazid similarly can also cause peripheral neuropathy. Compliance with medications and any relevant side effects should be checked, for example this can be particularly important in patients with epilepsy as ongoing epileptic seizures may be due to non-compliance or due to taking anticonvulsant medication at an inadequate dose.

Family history
Conditions with a genetic basis are relatively common in neurological practice (see Part III). It is therefore important to obtain a detailed family history. Furthermore, understanding the patient's fears about their symptoms or illness relies upon understanding of their prior exposure to and experiences of particular illnesses in their family.

Social history
Obtain history regarding smoking and drinking habits. This is relevant, for example peripheral neuropathy can occur in a patient with excessive alcohol drinking. Also detail exposure to illicit drugs and recent foreign or local travel. This may be relevant, for example in a patient with a lower motor neurone facial palsy who in preceding weeks suffered a tick bite while walking in a forest and now has neurological Lyme disease (neuroborreliosis).

Functional history
Understanding the level of disability or handicap a patient experiences due to an impairment (e.g. of arm function) is important in patients with long-term neurological conditions. One can work through a list of activities of daily living. Alternatively, one can work from head to toe asking the patient about specific functions, i.e. visual impairment, speech and swallowing impairment, upper limb impairment, impairment of bladder, bowel and sexual function and lower limb impairments, understanding along the way the consequences of these upon patient's occupation or on performance of activities of daily living and the impact on family/carers.

Systems review
Always review other body systems by means of direct questioning at the end of the history to pick up additional associated features of a systemic disturbance which may highlight the cause of a specific neurological symptom. As an example, a patient with nocturnal

breathlessness on lying flat may have neuromuscular and ventilatory impairment, which when considered with a history of weight loss, wasting and lack of sensory disturbance will point towards motor neurone disease.

Neurological examination

The typical clerking style of neurological examination performed by medical students and junior doctors includes the neurological examination of the head and neck (cranial nerve (CN) examination) as well as the upper and lower limbs. Additional routines of examination are also used to specifically test the cerebellar system, gait (see Chapter 11) and extrapyramidal system, domains of cognition or lobar functions of the brain (Table 3.1).

Suggested order of examination

General examination as a screening test including general inspection; mental status examination (not fully and formally undertaken on every neurological patient, however, may be important as neurological and psychiatric symptoms may coexist in illnesses such as dementia), including checking patient's appearance, behaviour, mood and for presence of delusions or hallucinations among others; higher mental function and speech; cranial nerves; upper and then lower limbs (inspection, tone and power); reflexes; sensory exam and finally coordination and gait.

Higher mental function and speech

Check patient's conscious level (using Glasgow Coma Scale as detailed in Appendix 2); orientation in time, place and person and finally perform a cognitive screening using abbreviated mental test score or mini-mental state examination if there is suspicion of cognitive impairment. Higher mental function may be impaired in various lobar syndromes, as detailed in Table 3.1. Note that 'apraxia' refers to the inability to perform an action despite an intact motor and sensory function while 'agnosia' refers to impaired perception despite the presence of an intact sensory function during neurological examination.

Check speech (usually assessed during obtaining history) for *dysphasia* syndromes (Table 3.1), including conduction dysphasia seen with lesions of the arcuate fasciculus (fibre tract connecting Broca's and Wernicke's area) and characterised mainly by impaired repetition; *dysarthria* implying difficulty with articulation by asking the patient to say, for example, 'British Constitution' (types include *cerebellar* characterised by slurred (drunk) and scanning speech, *spastic* as seen in pseudo-bulbar palsy in motor neurone disease and characterised by 'Donald Duck'-type voice, *monotonous* speech in extrapyramidal disease and *bulbar* speech in lower motor neurone syndromes like facial nerve palsy and characterised by nasal quality to speech) and *dysphonia* (impaired speech volume due to problem with respiratory muscles, for example myasthenia gravis).

Cranial nerves

For a detailed paper on the topic of 'cranial nerve examination', refer to Asghar and Abhinav 2011. Brief notes on examination of CN are as follows (Table 3.3):

- *I (Olfactory)*: Smell is not routinely tested unless patients complain of problem with smell; if needed, check ability of each nostril to distinguish different types of smell, including camphor, peppermint and others.
- *II (Optic)*: Each eye should be checked separately. Check acuity (Snellen chart), visual fields (to confrontation) and pupils (size, shape, reactivity to light, including direct and consensual response and accommodation) and perform a detailed opthalmoscopic examination inspecting the optic disc for papilloedema or atrophy.
- *III (Oculomotor), IV (trochlear), and VI (abducens)*: Check extraocular movements for full range of motion and evidence of diplopia, nystagmus, ptosis or internuclear opthalmoplegia (INO) (Chapter 18). Nystagmus refers to involuntary eye oscillations and can be normal at extreme lateral gaze. Direction of the fast phase should be noted; nystagmus can occur in the context of cerebellar or vestibular lesions. INO, for example, due to multiple sclerosis results due to a lesion in the medial longitudinal fasciculus and refers to failure of adduction of the ipsilateral eye with nystagmus in contralateral eye on abduction.

Table 3.3 Summary of signs and symptoms in cranial nerve lesions with their associated aetiology

Cranial nerve	Signs or symptoms of a lesion	Cause or lesion
I (Olfactory)	Change in sense of smell	Nasal obstruction
		Polyps or foreign bodies
		Viral infections
	Unable to identify common substances	Neurological causes
		Head injury
		Nasofrontal tumours
		Parkinson's disease
		Alzheimer's disease
II (Optic) (see Chapter 7)	Monocular blindness	Lesions of the eye
		Cataracts
		Intraocular haemorrhage
		Retinal detachments
		Diseases of the optic nerve
		Multiple sclerosis
		Tumours
	Bitemporal haemianopia	Compression of optic chiasm
		Pituitary tumour
	Homonymous haemianopia	Lesions of the optic tract
		Vascular lesions
		Neoplasm
		Optic radiation
		Lesions of the occipital lobe
	Visual inattention	Parietal lobe lesions
	Reduced visual fields	Glaucoma
		Chronic papilloedema

	Marcus Gunn Pupil (relative afferent pupillary defect) observed during the swinging flashlight test [patient's pupils constrict less (therefore appearing to dilate) when the light swings from the pupil of the unaffected eye to the pupil of the affected eye]	Damaged optic nerve pathway—indicating a decreased pupillary response to light in the affected eye (this detects less light than the functioning pathway)
	Constricted pupil	Horner's syndrome
		Opiate overdose
		Brainstem stroke
	Nystagmus	Physiological
		Congenital
		Visual impairment (difficulty in fixing gaze)
		Vestibular disease
		Cerebellar disease
	Papilloedema	Increased intracranial pressure
		Tumour
		Abscess
		Encephalitis
III (Oculomotor)	Divergent squint and diplopia (eyes down and out)	Paralysis of extraocular muscles (*superior rectus, inferior rectus and medial rectus*)
	Ptosis	Paralysis of levator palpebrae
		Horner's syndrome
		Myasthenia gravis
	Dilated pupil	Paralysis of sphincter pupillae
		Tumour
		Aneurysm
		Brainstem stroke

(continued)

Table 3.3 (*Continued*)

Cranial nerve	Signs or symptoms of a lesion	Cause or lesion
IV (Trochlear)	Eye elevation and outward rotation and diplopia (on looking down)	Paralysis of *superior oblique muscle*
		Tumour
		Aneurysm
V (Trigeminal)	Localised pain and vesicular eruption	Herpes zoster infection
	Anaesthesia and dissociated sensory loss	Syringobulbia
	Brisk jaw jerk	Bilateral upper motor neuron lesion
	Loss of corneal reflex, paralysed muscles of mastication (*deviation of jaw towards side of the lesion with unilateral lesion*) and loss of facial sensation	CN V palsy
		Neoplasm
		Infection
VI (Abducens)	Convergent squint and horizontal diplopia (with all movements excluding adduction)	Paralysis of *lateral rectus muscle*
		Tumour
		Aneurysm
VII (Facial)	Unilateral complete facial paralysis, hyperacusis, altered taste and impaired corneal reflex on affected side	Bell's palsy
	Unilateral lower facial palsy only (as forehead or frontalis has bilateral UMN innervations, so relative sparing of forehead is observed with unilateral UMN lesion)	UMN lesion
		Stroke
		Tumour
		MS
	Unilateral entire facial palsy (observed with LMN lesion where complete ipsilateral palsy with droopy mouth and loss of eyebrow lines and nasolabial folds is noted)	LMN lesion

		Stroke and tumour (acoustic neuroma)
		Ramsay Hunt syndrome
		Lyme disease, TB and HIV
		Diabetes and sarcoidosis
VIII (Auditory)	Conductive deafness	Ear disease
		Otitis externa or otitis media
		Paget's disease
		Perforated ear drum
	Sensorineural deafness	Congenital
		Acquired
		Presbycusis (ageing)
		Noise induced
		Ototoxicity (drugs)
	Attacks of dizziness and deafness	Acoustic neuroma (benign tumour). As it expands, it may compress adjacent CN V–VII
IX (Glossopharyngeal)	Altered sensation to palate and pharynx	CN IX palsy
		Base of skull tumour
		Stroke or trauma
X (Vagus)	Weak cough or dysphonia	Lesion of the recurrent laryngeal branch
	Asymmetrical soft palate (*with unilateral weakness palatal deviation towards the normal side*) and loss of gag reflex	CN X palsy
		Base of skull tumour
		Stroke or trauma
XI (Accessory)	Loss of power to sternocleidomastoid (SCM) or trapezius muscles	CN XI palsy

(*continued*)

Table 3.3 (*Continued*)

Cranial nerve	Signs or symptoms of a lesion	Cause or lesion
		Tumour
		Stroke
		Trauma
XII (Hypoglossal)	Tongue deviation (*towards side of lesion*) or weakness	Lower motor neuron lesion
	Tongue fasciculation	Motor neurone disease

Adapted from Asghar and Abhinav (2011).

- *V (Trigeminal)*: Check facial sensation (pinprick and light touch) in all three divisions (ophthalmic—V^1, maxillary—V^2 and mandibular—V^3), corneal reflex (CN V^1—afferent and CN VII—efferent) and motor function (CN V^3) by asking patient to open their mouth and clench in order to feel masseter and temporalis (muscles of mastication).
- *VII (Facial)*: Ask patient to raise eyebrows or look at the ceiling, puff up their cheeks or whistle and screw their eyes shut. Taste can also be checked in the anterior two-thirds of the tongue. Distinction between UMN type versus LMN type of facial nerve weaknesses is important (Table 3.3). Bell's palsy with its clinical features (as listed in Table 3.3) is a diagnosis of exclusion and typically has an abrupt onset with features of a unilateral LMN facial nerve palsy. Bell's phenomenon (inability to close eyes with rolling up of eye on attempted closure) may be seen. Short course of steroids (Prednisolone) may be tried with artificial tears and eye patch to protect the cornea.
- *VIII (Vestibulocochlear)*: Whisper a number while blocking the contralateral ear and ask patient to repeat the number. If there is unilateral hearing disturbance, carry out Weber's and Rinne's tests to distinguish between conductive and sensorineural hearing loss.
- *IX (Glossopharyngeal) and X (vagus)*: Ask patient to say 'Ahh' and look at the uvula for central elevation. Gag reflex (CN IX—afferent and CN X—efferent) may be checked.
- *XI (Accessory)*: Ask patient to shrug their shoulders (trapezius) or turn head to one side against resistance (sternocleidomastoid).
- *XII (Hypoglossal)*: Check for fasciculation and wasting with tongue inside mouth (LMN lesion). Ask the patient to move it from side to side checking for any slowing of the tongue movement (UMN lesion).

Upper and lower limbs

Typically start with inspection and then examine tone and power. Tendon reflexes, sensation and finally coordination and gait are also tested.

Specifically inspect for muscle wasting or atrophy (in LMN syndromes) and fasciculations (e.g. in motor neurone disease) and observe the posture (e.g. stooped posture of Parkinson's) and check for presence of any abnormal movements, for example tremor (see Chapter 20). Check for *pyramidal drift* (pronation and drifting down of outstretched arms) occurring for example with UMN lesions in corticospinal tract.

Tone

Testing tone can help determine whether the lesion is within the central or peripheral nervous system. Tone may be increased, decreased (hypotonia) or normal and is best assessed at wrist, elbow, hip and knee. If increased, it can be either in spastic or rigid fashion. Lesions

Table 3.4 Muscle strength grading (MRC scale)

Grade	Muscle strength
0	No contraction
1	Flicker of contraction
2	Movement with elimination of gravity
3	Active movement against gravity
4	Active movement against resistance (4− slight, 4 moderate and 4+ strong)
5	Normal power

affecting the corticospinal tract (UMN) produce a spastic increase in tone, best elicited by a rapid flexion extension movement of the elbow where a so-called spastic catch or a sudden increase in tone may be felt. In contrast, a rigid increase (increased through a whole range of movement) in tone typically localises to problems within the basal ganglia (extrapyramidal system, for example Parkinson's disease) and is best elicited either by a slow flexion extension movement at the elbow, knees or ankles or by a slow circling movement at the wrist. Rigidity may be described as 'lead pipe' and when combined with breaks or tremors as being 'cogwheeling'. Rigidity may be heightened by asking the patient to perform movement of the contralateral limb (synkinesis).

Power testing
Power testing involves assessing power in a given muscle group around each joint. For example at the elbow, power is assessed for elbow flexion and extension. Power testing is documented using the Medical Research Council (MRC) grading scale shown in Table 3.4. Always compare with the strength on the contralateral side.

It is important to be aware of the muscle groups being tested along with innervating nerve roots and named nerves (Table 3.5).

Reflexes
Reflex (segmental levels in Table 3.5) testing requires practice and reflexes may be absent, decreased, normal, increased and finally increased with clonus (contraction of muscle when stretched and tested for at the ankle and quantified in terms of number of beats). Increased reflexes are associated with a lesion in the UMN pathway (corticospinal tract) whereas decreased or absent reflexes occur with a problem in the peripheral nervous system (LMN pathway) with a loss of a reflex or reflexes being due to failure of either the afferent (sensory) or the efferent (motor) arm of the reflex arc. The plantar response is assessed using stimulus on lateral sole with an upgoing or extensor plantar or Babinski sign (associated with UMN lesions within the corticospinal tract) being defined as extension of big toe with fanning out or spreading out of other toes. Normal response is flexion of the toes.

Note on UMN versus LMN lesions
- LMN lesions lead to hypotonia, hyporeflexia or areflexia; fasciculations with atrophy of the affected muscles therefore causing a flaccid paralysis on the same side and at the level of the lesion.
- UMN lesions lead to hypertonicity, hyperreflexia with or without clonus, Babinski sign, loss of abdominal and cremasteric reflex and disuse atrophy. UMN lesions always lead to spastic weakness which is below the level of the lesion and could be ipsilateral (if lesion affects corticospinal tract in spinal cord) or contralateral (if lesion is between the cerebral cortex and medulla above the pyramidal decussation).

Table 3.5 Important muscle groups and spinal nerve roots with reflexes for upper and lower limbs

Segment	Muscle	Action	Nerve	Reflex
C5, C6	Deltoid	Abduct arm	Axillary	
C5, C6	Biceps	Elbow flexion	Musculocutaneous	Biceps
C5, **C6**	Brachioradialis	Forearm flexion with thumb up	Radial	Supinator
C6, **C7**, C8	Triceps	Elbow extension	Radial	Triceps
C6, C7	Extensor carpi radialis	Wrist extension	Radial	
C7, C8	Extensor digitorum	Finger extension	Posterior interosseous (branch of radial nerve)	
C7, **C8**, T1	Flexor digitorum profundus (ulnar part)	Flexion of distal phalanx of fingers (4 and 5)	Ulnar	
C7, **C8**, T1	Flexor digitorum profundus (radial part)	Flexion of distal phalanx of fingers (2 and 3)	Anterior interosseous (branch of median nerve)	
C8, **T1**	Interossei	Abduct fingers	Ulnar	
C8, **T1**	Abductor pollicis brevis	Thumb abduction	Median	
C8, **T1**	Opponens pollicis	Thumb opposition	Median	
L1, L2	Iliopsoas	Hip flexion	Lumbosacral plexus	
L5, S1	Gluteus maximus	Hip extension	Inferior gluteal	
L3, L4	Quadriceps	Knee extension	Femoral	Knee
L5, **S1**	Hamstrings	Knee flexion	Sciatic	
L4, **L5**	Tibialis anterior	Ankle dorsiflexion	Deep peroneal (branch of common peroneal nerve)	
L5, S1	Extensor hallucis longus	Great toe extension	Deep peroneal	
S1, S2	Gastrocnemius	Ankle plantarflexion	Tibial (branch of sciatic)	Ankle
L5, S1	Peroneus longus and brevis	Foot eversion	Superficial peroneal (branch of common peroneal nerve)	
L5, S1	Posterior tibialis	Foot inversion	Tibial	

Major innervations indicated in bold.

Sensory

Different modalities of sensation are conveyed by different pathways (see Figure 2.3) and each should be assessed. Always teach the test first prior to carrying it out.

Dorsal column (fine touch, joint position and vibration sense on ipsilateral side)
Vibration sense is assessed with 128 Hz tuning fork; start with sternum to familiarise patient with the vibration sense and then apply to bony prominences (including base of big toe, medial malleolus, knee and elbow) starting distally. If sensation is normal distally, there is no need to carry out tests more proximally.

Test for joint position sense is taught with patient's eyes open followed by movement of the joint with patient's eyes closed and asking them regarding the direction of movement of the joint, i.e. up or down.

Light touch is tested using cotton wool or fingertip in all dermatomes (Figure 3.1), including those in the affected ones.

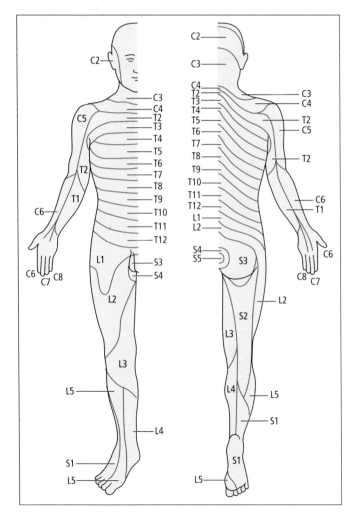

Figure 3.1 Dermatomes represented on anterior and posterior aspects of the body.

Spinothalamic tract (pain and temperature sensation on contralateral side)
Pain (tested using pinprick) sensation is tested in all dermatomes (Figure 3.1) including those in the affected ones with patient's eyes closed. Teach the patient first by applying the pin in a normal area of skin.

Temperature sensation is not tested routinely; however, it can be carried out using test tubes with hot and cold water. With sensory losses (see Chapter 10), always map out the area and distribution, for example glove and stocking distribution with diabetic peripheral neuropathy (see Chapter 24).

Gait and coordination
Gait assessment with associated disturbances is covered in detail in Chapter 11. In brief, ask patient to walk normally followed by heel to toe test (indicates ataxia if patient is unable to perform the test). Romberg's test (patient stands with their feet together followed by eyes closed) is positive if patients lose their balance with eyes closed and indicates posterior column pathology (joint position dysfunction leading to sensory ataxia). If unable to do this with eyes open, cerebellar ataxia may be implied (however, not Romberg's positive). Note that Romberg's test is useful for distinguishing between cerebellar and sensory ataxia in a patient with a broad-based gait.

Coordination is typically tested with finger to nose test; heel–shin testing and using repeated movements (rapid pronation and supination of hand on dorsum of other hand; impairment with this is referred to as *dysdiadochokinesis* and occurs with cerebellar pathology).

Reference
Asghar R, Abhinav K (2011) Cranial nerve examination. *International Journal of Clinical Skills* **5** (1): 56–63.

4 Neurological investigations

Neurophysiology

Electroencephalogram (EEG)

- Used for recording the electrical activity of the brain via electrodes attached to the scalp.
- Principal use of EEG is in the diagnosis and management of different seizure disorders with the EEG being performed during ictal and interictal phases.
- Can be recorded with video monitoring.
- Diagnostic yield can be increased with the use of forced hyperventilation (e.g. triggering spike and wave activity), photic stimulation, sleep deprivation and repeating the EEG.
- While interpreting interictal EEG, background rhythm and paroxysmal changes need to be considered. Normal background rhythm is called 'alpha' at 8–13 Hz (mainly in the occipital lobes when one is awake and quiet). Slowing of the background rhythm can occur in metabolic encephalopathy (renal and hepatic failure), drug overdose and other degenerative conditions.
- Paroxysmal changes (spikes <70 ms, sharp waves: 70–200 ms) can be focal (suggesting a structural lesion) or generalised. Generalised spike and wave activity at 3 Hz is seen in absence seizures (Table 4.1).

> Remember: A normal interictal EEG does not exclude the diagnosis of epilepsy. A high proportion of patients with epilepsy may have a normal interictal EEG. Although specific, EEG has low sensitivity for diagnosing epilepsy.

- Ictal EEG is ideal for diagnosing epilepsy. During a generalised tonic–clonic seizure, high-voltage synchronised discharges of 100 µV are seen. Continuous video EEG monitoring to localise a seizure focus is used as part of preoperative evaluation for surgical treatment of medically refractory epilepsy.
- Other uses include non-convulsive status, confirming brain death (not essential) and burst suppression.
- Memorise these characteristic EEG changes (Table 4.1) frequently featuring in examinations.

Evoked potential studies

- These assess the sensory pathways from the sensory organ to the cerebral cortex, for example visual (VEP), brain stem auditory (BSAEP) and somatosensory (SSEP) evoked potentials.
- Stimuli, for example clicking noise for BSAEP, are delivered while recordings are made from scalp electrodes.
- A delay in the potential implies demyelination while a reduction in amplitude suggests axonal degeneration.
- A delayed VEP may be due to a subclinical lesion of MS affecting the optic pathway. Similarly, delayed BSAEP may occur in the context of acoustic neuroma or MS.
- SSEP involves assessing posterior column pathway of the sensory system. Painless electrical stimulation is applied at different points, for example above the clavicle or the lumbar and cervical spine with simultaneous recording from contralateral parietal sensory cortex.
- An abnormal SSEP can therefore occur with MS or spinal cord lesions. Intraoperative SSEP is useful during spinal surgery. A drop in amplitude intraoperatively may signify neural damage.

nical conditions of note with characteristic EEG changes

	EEG changes
	3 Hz spike and wave
West syndrome	Interictal hypsarrhythmia
Juvenile myoclonic epilepsy	Polyspike discharges
Creutzfeldt–Jakob disease	Bilateral sharp waves (1.5–2 Hz, later triphasic); can occur with simultaneous myoclonic jerks
Herpes simplex encephalitis	Bilateral periodic lateralizing epileptiform discharges (regular sharp waves with background slow activity)
Metabolic encephalopathy	Generalised slow activity
Subacute sclerosing panencephalitis	Body jerks and associated periodic high voltage

- Transcranial motor evoked potentials involves electrical stimulation of motor cortex with a recording of potentials from muscle. This again can be useful for surgery of the spinal cord.

Nerve conduction studies (NCS)
- Assesses motor and sensory functions of myelinated fibres in terms of two principal measurements, conduction velocity and amplitude.
- Motor element of NCS involves stimulation of motor nerve at two points (distal and proximal) and recording the amplitude of the compound muscle action potential (CMAP) at a fixed different point. The sensory element involves stimulation at one point with recording the potential at a different distant site.
- Conduction velocity is measured using the distance and the latency.
- Axonal disease (e.g. diabetic neuropathy) leads to normal velocity motor conduction with reduced amplitude while demyelinating disease, for example Guillain–Barré syndrome, increases the latency thereby decreasing the conduction velocity.

> Remember: The point about the delay versus the decrease in amplitude seen in association with demyelinating versus axonal degeneration, respectively.

Other parameters measured include H reflex and F response.

Electromyography (EMG)
- Involves insertion of a needle electrode into muscle and observing the electrical activity as well as listening to the auditory signal.
- A motor unit refers to a single alpha-motor neuron and all the corresponding muscle fibres innervated by it. A motor unit potential (MUP) is triphasic.
- After a normal insertional activity related to insertion of the needle, spontaneous activity is assessed. Resting muscle is silent or has brief monophasic negative potentials. Fibrillation potential (not observed through the skin) due to a single-fibre activity is a triphasic potential related to denervation, for example in ALS, poliomyelitis

and inflammatory muscle disease, for example polymyositis. Fasciculation potential in comparison is related to discharge of motor unit (group of fibres) and can be observed through the skin. This is seen in association with ALS, poliomyelitis and hypocalcaemia among others.

- Smooth contraction of the muscle leads to an interference pattern with recruitment of motor units. Consequently, the shape, size and frequency of resulting MUPs are analysed. Denervation is associated with decreased amplitude of MUPs with increased duration and a polyphasic pattern while myopathy in comparison is associated with decreased duration and amplitude.
- In myasthenia gravis (MG), a decremental response or a decrease in the amplitude of the CMAP is observed with repetitive nerve stimulation of a motor nerve; single-fibre EMG shows increased 'jitter'. This contrasts with an incremental response or an increase in amplitude observed in Lambert–Eaton myasthenic syndrome (LEMS).

Remember: Decremental versus incremental response in MG versus LEMS, respectively.

Neuroradiology

Computed tomography (CT) (see CT images throughout the book)
- Most available neuroimaging technique.
- Appearance described in terms of 'density', i.e. hyperdense or hypodense.
- High density is related to a higher Hounsfield unit (HU). Hounsfield units define the extent of attenuation of the X-ray beam on CT scan.
- Bone therefore has a HU of +600, CSF has a HU of +5 and fresh blood has a HU of 75–80. CSF will therefore be hypodense in comparison to blood and bone. Similarly, blood is hyperdense in comparison to brain parenchyma (with a HU between 20 and 40 units) (refer to Chapter 33 for details on CT appearance of different stages of subdural haematoma).
- Useful and ideal for cases of intracerebral and subarachnoid haemorrhage, traumatic contusions and haematomas, for example extradural and subdural collections and bony injury including depressed skull fracture.
- Limited role in spinal pathology and contraindicated in pregnancy unless performed as an emergency investigation.
- Iodinated water-soluble intravenous contrast agents (caution: risk of anaphylaxis and allergic reactions) are used in certain circumstances, for example in cerebral abscess, tumours, subdural empyema, and so on to elicit contrast enhancement.

Magnetic Resonance Imaging (MRI)
- Does not involve ionising radiation.
- Contraindicated in patients with pacemakers, ferromagnetic aneurysm clips, metallic implants and metallic fragments within the eye. Also, relatively contraindicated during the first trimester of pregnancy leading to miscarriage.
- Lesions are described in terms of signal intensity (hypertense versus hypointense).
- Ideal for imaging CNS tumours, posterior fossa lesions, demyelinating disease, for example MS plaques and in the spinal cord for demonstrating disc herniation and neural compromise. Gadolinium is used as a contrast agent for demonstrating enhancement with tumours and abscesses.
- *T1 weighted image (T1WI)*: Good anatomical detail visualised (Figure 4.1). The following are hyperintense (white) on T1WI: fat, melanin, and blood (>48 h–14 days). CSF is characteristically dark. Majority of pathology is hypointense.
- *T2 weighted image (T2WI)*: The sequence of choice for highlighting pathology which is usually hyperintense including cerebral oedema. CSF is characteristically bright while

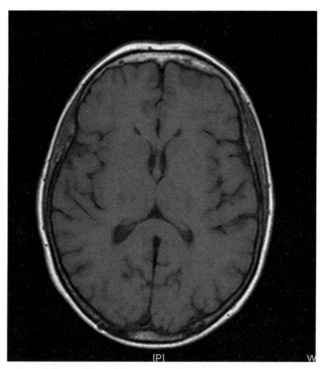

Figure 4.1 T1WI axial image of the brain (note CSF is dark).

bone and fat are dark (Figure 4.2). Acute (1–3 days) and early subacute (>3 to ≤7 days) blood is hypointense while blood (7–14 days) is hyperintense.

> *Remember: CSF signal intensity can be used to determine the type of sequence, i.e. hypointense in T1WI compared to hyperintense in T2WI. Bone is dark in both. Interpretation of blood on MRI scan is complex with varying signal intensities depending on the age of the clot and its breakdown product.*

- STIR sequences combine T1 and T2 suppressing signal from fat. Used in spinal pathology.
- Diffusion-weighted imaging and perfusion-weighted imaging are used in patients with suspected ischaemic brain injury.
- Magnetic resonance spectroscopy relies on spectroscopy of other molecules and atoms besides hydrogen, thereby providing information on chemistry of specific lesions like tumours or abscess. One use for example is in differentiating between the two aforementioned using choline and lactate peaks.
- MRI can also be applied to delineate arterial (MR angiogram, for example used in screening for aneurysms, neck vessel dissection) or venous anatomy (MR venogram, for example used in suspected cases of venous sinus thrombosis).

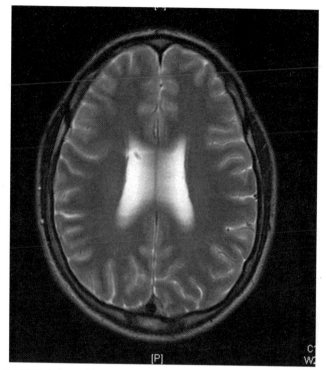

Figure 4.2 T2WI axial image of the brain (note CSF is bright).

Angiography
- Catheter angiogram remains the gold standard for imaging intra- and extracranial vessels.
- Local anaesthetic/sedation is used prior to the insertion of the catheter into the femoral artery and then into the carotid or vertebral artery origin with the help of an image intensifier. Computerised digital subtraction angiography technique is performed.
- The main indications are for diagnosing cerebral aneurysms or arteriovenous malformations in cases of suspected subarachnoid haemorrhage. Interventional angiography involving coiling of the aneurysm is being increasingly used in the treatment of aneurysms (see Figure 16.2).
- Risk of a resulting permanent neurological deficit is about 0.1%.

Lumbar puncture and CSF analysis
- A widely used investigation in neurological and neurosurgical practice. Indications include suspected meningitis of bacterial, viral or fungal aetiology; CNS demyelinating conditions like MS and peripheral demyelinating neuropathy, for example GBS and in cases of suspected SAH with a normal CT scan.
- In adults, intercristal line (line connecting the superior border of the iliac crests) passes through the spine at L4 spinous process or between L4 and L5 spinous processes. The recommendation is to use L4 and L5 interspace or a level higher (L3 and L4).

*r: Although the dural sac extends to S2, spinal cord terminates at the level of
 ral bodies of L1 and L2; therefore, if correctly performed at an appropriate
level, should not damage the spinal cord.*

Place patient in a left lateral position, with the shoulders square and pillow under the head
and between the knees. Ideally a 22G needle with stylet *in situ* (under a strict aseptic technique and following infiltration of a local anaesthetic) is inserted aiming slightly cranially (or
towards the umbilicus).

- The layers traversed through include skin, subcutaneous tissue, supra and then interspi-
nous ligaments, ligamentum flavum, epidural space and then through the dura and
arachnoid into the subarachnoid space. Removal of stylet will lead to a flow of CSF.
Using a three-way tap, measure the opening pressure and collect samples in at least
three tubes: microscopy, cell count, culture, sensitivity and gram stain; protein, glucose
and oligoclonal bands (on electrophoresis); cytology for the presence of malignant cells
(e.g. in carcinomatous meningitis). Closing pressure should be measured if the opening
pressure was raised followed by reinsertion of stylet and withdrawal of the needle. A
blood sample should be taken at the same time for blood glucose, protein and oligoclonal bands (e.g. if diagnosis of MS suspected) (Table 4.2).

Table 4.2 Different clinical conditions with their characteristic CSF findings

Clinical condition	Opening pressure (cm H_2O)	Cells (mm^3)	Protein (mg/dL)	Glucose	Comments
Normal	7–18	<5 (Lymphocytes)	<45	50% of serum glucose	
Acute bacterial meningitis	Raised	>5–20,000 (polymorphs)	Raised (100–1000)	<30–40%	Cloudy/turbid appearance
TB meningitis	Raised	50–500 (Initially polymorph and then lymphocytic)	Raised (up to 700)	<40%	Similar findings in fungal meningitis, positive Ziehl–Neelsen test, TB PCR, culture may take 6–8 weeks
Viral meningitis/ encephalitis	Normal	>5–200 (Lymphocytes)	Normal or raised (up to 100)	Normal	CSF PCR for herpes simplex virus
Multiple sclerosis	Normal	Normal-up to 50 (lymphocytes)	Normal or raised (up to 100, usually <55)	Normal	Protein electrophoresis of CSF shows oligoclonal bands in CSF but not in serum
Guillain–Barré	Normal	Normal	Raised (>55)	Normal	'Albuminocytological dissociation', i.e. raised protein without elevated cell count

Important for the exam!

- Patient can lay flat for an hour or so after the procedure.
- Complications of the procedure include headache (commonest and due to low intra-cranial pressure; usually resolves spontaneously and risk reduced with the use of smaller needles, for example 22G; advise bed rest; hydration; analgesia and caffeine intake with epidural blood patch for refractory cases), infection (meningitis), transient radicular pain due to nerve root impingement (change trajectory towards contralateral side), spinal extradural haematoma in coagulopathic patients and acute tonsillar herniation.

Remember: To obtain imaging to exclude an intracranial mass lesion or obstructive hydrocephalus in patients with impaired consciousness or focal neurological deficits or papilloedema prior to performing an LP due to the risk of acute tonsillar herniation.

- In cases of suspected traumatic tap (due to injury to venous plexus), CSF sample should be collected in four bottles and unlike SAH, red cell count will reduce with successive bottles and xanthochromia will be absent (see Chapter 16). A failed LP (due to severe degenerative spine disease or obesity) may be followed up with a request to perform the procedure under image intensifier guidance.
- Contraindications include suspected or confirmed intracranial mass lesion or obstructive hydrocephalus, sepsis or infection at the area of LP, for example sacral sores, and coagulopathy (low platelet count, impaired clotting profile or patients on anticoagulants).

Part II
Complaints: Face-to-face with the patient

5   Headache

Commonest reasons for referral to general neurology clinics:
- Commonly due to one of the primary headache disorders but may be secondary in origin due to a potential life-threatening aetiology.
- Acute headaches or marked exacerbation of long-standing headaches can present as an emergency.
- Chronic headaches tend to present as recurrent attendances at the community physicians.
- A comprehensive history, particularly the history of the presenting complaint, is crucial for correct diagnosis.

Useful selected questions to ask/facts to establish?
- *History of the presenting complaint:* Start with an open question, for example 'tell me about your headache,' and allow the patient to speak freely until they stop. Follow with targeted questions.
- *Number of types of headache experienced by the patient:* Ask directly about the number of different types of headache. Typically ranges from one to several. Understanding, for example, that a patient is suffering frequent tension-type headaches with intermittent migraine-type headaches is important as not all recurrent headaches in a single patient will have the same cause.

> *Remember: Patients with chronic headache disorders remain at the same risk as the background population for developing life-threatening new headache conditions such as subarachnoid haemorrhage or brain tumour.*

Having established the number of types of headache, the following questions can be asked for each subtype:
- *Duration:* Establish the duration of headache (e.g. a hyperacute onset of headache raising the alarm for a possible vascular aetiology, for example subarachnoid haemorrhage (SAH)) with an accurate and prompt diagnosis being life saving; headaches for the first time and progressing over days or weeks may be due to infective causes (meningitis/encephalitis) or inflammatory (giant cell arteritis) and finally headaches going back many years are typically benign and primary in origin.
- Establish whether continuous or episodic.
- If episodic, establish the frequency, periodicity and duration of the episodes.
- If continuous, establish whether constant or waxing and waning in severity and, if waxing and waning, when these changes occur, for how long they last and the exacerbating and relieving factors.
- If episodic, in which part of the head does the pain start? Nature of the pain, i.e. throbbing, pulsatile or stabbing? Evolution of the pain, i.e. does it remain localised to one area, spread to involve one half of the head or become generalised?
- Is the headache feature-full or featureless? (Migraine-type headaches, for example, are feature-full with associated nausea, vomiting and photophobia whereas tension-type headaches are usually featureless with headache and possibly associated posterior neck ache being the only symptoms).
- Symptoms that precede headache onset [(e.g. visual disturbance including flashing lights (tycopsia), zigzag lines, fortification spectra and spreading haemianopia in migraine-type headache)].

- If any associated features (e.g. in migraine, nausea, vomiting, photophobia, phonophobia, dizziness, unilateral sensory disturbance including pins and needles).
- Time period for the headache to reach its maximum severity (e.g. in SAH, usually over seconds to a minute whereas in migraine, typically many minutes to an hour, except in specific circumstances such as migraine variants including coital cephalalgia or exertional headache).
- If any triggers for the headaches (lack of sleep or excessive sleep, alcohol or certain foodstuffs in migraine).
- If any exacerbating factors (e.g. a new onset of continuous headache progressively worsening over weeks to months exacerbated by cough or physical strain and worse in the morning may suggest raised intracranial pressure secondary to an intracranial mass; migraine in women during/with menstruation).
- If any relieving factors (including both pharmacological and behavioural factors such as lying quietly in a darkened room or sleeping in migraine).
- If any pain in the face (e.g. severe unilateral ocular pain occurring in males in the early hours of the morning suggesting cluster headache or lightening-type unilateral facial pains triggered by chewing or eating suggesting a diagnosis of trigeminal neuralgia).
- Ask further specific targeted questions regarding suspected diagnosis (e.g. with cluster headache ask about unilateral eye tearing, unilateral nasal stuffiness or unilateral nose running; with giant cell arteritis ask about unilateral scalp tenderness, pain on hair brushing, jaw claudication and chest pain).
- Past medical history (systemic medical conditions can present with headache, for example severe anaemia and metabolic disturbances including alterations in sodium, calcium or glucose).
- History of medications (e.g. ones used for headache relief acutely and those taken as prophylactic agents, for example in migraine or cluster headache).
- Careful family history (e.g. a strong family history of migraine).

Remember that one of the common causes of persistent featureless headaches presenting to the physician is analgesic overuse headache. This is an important diagnosis as the treatment is reduction and withdrawal of medications provoking and maintaining the headache rather than more tablets.

Other points to consider
- A careful neurological examination looking for evidence of localising signs secondary to a focal intracranial disturbance (e.g. raised intracranial pressure may produce optic disc swelling in addition to false localising signs (Chapter 30); with suspected meningitis signs of meningeal irritation, for example neck stiffness, photophobia and Kernig's sign may be present).
- Full general medical examination, as headaches may be secondary to systemic illness.

Differential diagnoses (see Chapter 12)

Basic investigations
- *Baseline*: Blood tests (e.g. FBC for anaemia, infection; U & E for evidence of metabolic disturbance or renal disturbance; LFT).
- *Imaging*: With suspected structural, infective or vascular cause, prompt brain imaging should be performed, either an initial CT (e.g. with suspected subarachnoid haemorrhage) or MRI if more appropriate.
- Lumbar puncture (LP) may be required (Chapter 4 for further details) in suspected cases with SAH, meningitis, encephalitis or idiopathic intracranial hypertension. With CT negative suspected SAH cases, analyse CSF for haem pigments, including oxyhaemoglobin and bilirubin (Chapter 16 for further details).

Remember: Obtain imaging to exclude an intracranial mass lesion or obstructive hydrocephalus in patients with impaired consciousness or focal neurological deficits or papilloedema prior to performing an LP due to the risk of acute tonsillar herniation, which results in permanent neurological disability or death.

Basic management
Depends upon the underlying cause and discussed in Part III in relevant chapters.

Blackouts

A very common presentation:
- Important to realise the non-specific nature of this complaint.
- Always obtain an accurate history from both the patient and the witness if available.
  Two most important differentials (Table 6.1):
- *Syncope* (commoner)
- *Seizures*

> *Remember: If recovery from cerebral hypoperfusion is delayed in a syncopal event (e.g. by keeping patient upright), secondary anoxic convulsions (provoked seizures) can occur.*

Useful selected questions to ask/facts to establish (syncope versus seizures)

In general, ascertain the details of the events prior, during and following an attack.

> *Remember: Always ask about any previous episodes and loss of consciousness (LOC) and take a full collateral history from a witness if available.*

Prior to attack

Any warning signs?
- Brief warning (aura) of epilepsy, for example strange smell or taste or feeling, for example rising epigastric sensation.
- Prodromal symptoms preceding syncope, for example light-headedness, visual dimming and feeling sweaty.
- Any identifiable triggers/provoking factors? [(Emotional response (seeing blood), hyperventilation, prolonged standing and hot surroundings in vasovagal syncope; immediately

Table 6.1 Clinical conditions leading to blackouts with points to note

Clinical conditions	Points to note
Syncope	See above
Epilepsy (tonic–clonic and complex partial) (Chapter 17)	See above
Hypoglycaemia	Seen particularly in diabetics. Light-headedness and autonomic changes, for example tremor, pallor, sweating and tachycardia precede LOC
Transient ischaemic attacks (TIAs) (Chapter 13)	TIAs rarely lead to blackouts
Migraine (Chapter 12)	Syncope can occur during a migraine attack
Drop attacks	A benign condition unless secondary to hydrocephalus; patient, more commonly an elderly lady, suddenly drops to the ground without warning and LOC. Resolves spontaneously after a number of attacks

post voiding urine in micturition syncope; standing up in postural hypotension; or alcoholic binge or abrupt withdrawal and head injury in seizure).]

During the attack
- Posture, for example lying down or standing? (Vasovagal syncope is very unusual if patient is lying down).
- Patient awake or asleep during event? (Seizures often arise from sleep).
- Any loss of consciousness? (Both seizures and syncope can cause this).
- Duration of loss of consciousness? (Seconds in syncope versus minutes in seizures).
- Still while unconscious (more suggestive of syncope) or stiffness followed by jerking of limbs? (Tonic–clonic seizures)
- Involuntarily passing of urine or faeces? (Considered to be a seizure marker but can occur in syncope).
- Biting of tongue? (Rare in syncope; commoner in tonic–clonic seizures, where often the side of the tongue is damaged).
- Any other associated symptoms like palpitations or breathlessness? (Arrhythmias in cardiac syncope)

After the attack
- Period of confusion, amnesia or drowsiness after attack? [Rapid recovery in syncope without prolonged confusion or amnesia versus prolonged drowsiness and confusion in epileptic seizures (postictal period)]

> *Remember: Take a full detailed medical history including past medical history (e.g. cardiac problems (syncope more likely); previous meningitis, encephalitis, head injury, stroke (seizure more likely) or diabetes); drug history (e.g. antihypertensives); family history and social history, including alcohol and recreational drug abuse.*

Differential diagnoses (Table 6.1)
- Others—Subarachnoid haemorrhage (sudden severe headache with possible loss of consciousness), hyperventilation and panic attacks, pseudo-seizures (non-epileptic attacks) and choking.

Basic investigations

> *Remember: Carry out a thorough cardiac and neurological examination prior to requesting investigations.*

Carotid sinus massage (with monitoring) and measurement of postural blood pressure should be performed, if indicated for carotid sinus hypersensitivity and orthostatic hypotension respectively, especially in the elderly. A definitely syncopal event, for example vasovagal or micturition syncope, may not need further investigations.

In a *syncopal* attack, consider the following tests:
- Postural blood pressure.
- *Bloods*: FBC, U & E, fasting glucose.
- ECG initially followed by 24 h ECG, echocardiogram and a tilt table test if indicated.
  If seizure suspected, check routine bloods as above and further consider the following:
- EEG (sleep-deprived EEG has higher sensitivity).
- MRI/CT scan to investigate for space-occupying lesion acting as seizure focus.

Basic management
Depends on the underlying pathology. Advise to refrain from driving until a cause determined, and then as applicable.

7   Visual disturbances

This chapter follows a different format from the rest of the chapters in Part II owing to the nature of the topic.

Loss of vision

Visual loss may be due to a problem within the eye, the optic nerve or the posterior visual pathways.

[handwritten annotations: painless decline in VA, acute vs chronic-tunnel vision, Blurry, Colour/nighttime, peripheral scotoma, & care, halos, arcuate, Short vs long, nighttime vision]

Local eye disease

- Disturbance of the eye and vision is common and it is important to consider local changes within the eye.
- Consider corneal damage, cataract, refractive errors, glaucoma and retinal disturbance.
- Correct a refractive error producing myopia with a pinhole early in the course of considering the cause of visual loss. Having excluded the causes of visual disturbance from the surface of the eye back to the retina, consider neurological dysfunction of the optic nerve or posterior visual pathways.

[handwritten: Neuritis; SOL, stroke, CCA]

Optic nerve disturbance

- Optic nerve lesions cause a disturbance of central vision (scotoma) with a reduction in visual acuity (Figure 7.1).
- Visual loss due to anterior lesions of the optic nerve reduces visual acuity leading to reduced perception of distant objects and potential difficulty with reading.

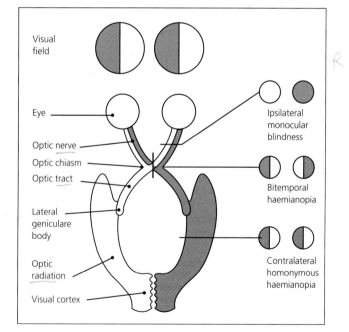

Figure 7.1 Visual field defect according to the location of the lesion along the visual pathway.

- Determine the loss of acuity: test in either eye separately for central vision using, for example, a Snellen chart.
- Understanding the temporal onset of central visual loss is often the most useful determinant in recognising the aetiology of anterior optic nerve disturbance.
- Determining whether central visual loss is episodic (and if so, of what duration) or persistent is further discriminating.

Optic nerve disturbance causing sudden onset of transient visual loss

- Sudden onset of unilateral visual loss may be vascular in origin due to disturbance in the ophthalmic artery (amaurosis fugax). Often a falling or rising curtain affecting either the upper or lower half of the vision from one eye due to occlusion of either the superior or the inferior ophthalmic artery is described. Hence, so-called altitudinal defects often reflect a vascular aetiology.
- Amaurosis fugax is a transient ischaemic episode of the ophthalmic artery and typically occurs in older patients with vascular risk factors.
- Sudden temporary central visual loss also occurs with so-called obscurations of vision secondary to raised intracranial pressure.
- Such visual obscurations are typically very brief, lasting seconds to minutes only. Visual obscurations are normally seen where background intracranial pressure is high, for whatever reason, and then with a provoking manoeuvre (such as coughing or straining) which raises intracranial pressure further causing brief visual loss. With visual obscurations, look for swollen discs.
- Transient episodic visual loss can occur with previous optic neuritis (demyelination/ multiple sclerosis) when the patient's body temperature rises, such as with exercise, the so-called Uhthoff's phenomena.

Optic nerve disturbance causing persistent visual loss

- Persistent visual loss may be acute, subacute or chronic in its progression.
- Acute (occurring over minutes) persistent visual loss is often due to a vascular aetiology affecting the ophthalmic arteries or veins.
- Subacute relapsing remitting central visual loss is commonly due to inflammation/ demyelination within the optic nerves, such as is seen in multiple sclerosis.
- Subacute and chronic progressive central visual loss may be due to a compressive structural cause and requires urgent MRI imaging. Lesions compressing the optic nerve are frequently benign but prompt intervention remains important to preserve vision.
- If a structural cause has been ruled out, toxic (tobacco/alcohol), nutritional (B1/B12), drug-induced and hereditary optic neuropathies (Leber's optic neuropathy) should be considered.

> Remember: Acute bilateral visual loss due to optic nerve damage may be seen due to toxicity, such as following ingestion of methanol.

Disturbance of the posterior visual pathways

- Disturbance of the visual pathways at the optic chiasm, optic radiations or in the occipital cortex typically produce loss of vision in one quarter or one half of the visual field (haemianopia) (Figure 7.1).
- In the posterior visual pathway disturbance, visual acuity may be preserved whereas visual field perception is reduced in the affected opposite visual field.

Diplopia (double vision)

- A common cause of visual disturbance presenting to the general practitioner or neurologist.
- Peripheral or central in origin. Peripheral causes include disturbance of the extraocular muscles, the neuromuscular junction (myasthenia gravis) and the third, fourth and sixth

cranial nerves. Central causes include disturbances of eye movements initiated and co-ordinated by brainstem nuclei.

- During assessment, it is important to determine the effect of covering either eye.
- Determine whether the images are horizontally or vertically separated.
- Determine the effect of gaze direction on the separation of the dual images. Check for ptosis and proptosis and determine pupil size and the range of eye movements.

8   Dizziness and vertigo

'Giddiness' or 'dizziness' can be used by patients to mean a variety of sensations:
- Important to distinguish symptoms of vestibular dysfunction from non-vestibular symptoms, for example postural syncope (giddiness on standing up) versus unsteadiness related to cerebellar/brainstem pathology.
- Vertigo is defined as an illusion of movement of the patient and his/her environment (rotatory or non-rotatory). The sense of abnormal movement or disequilibrium is felt in the patient's head and may take the form of the room spinning; the floor rising or a sensation of swaying or moving up and down as if on a boat.
- Vertigo can be of peripheral (disorders of labyrinth or vestibular nerve) origin or of central (brainstem) origin.

Useful selected questions to ask/facts to establish?
- Establish whether symptoms are consistent with a vertiginous episode, as above?
- Duration of the episode (e.g. vertigo due to benign positional vertigo (BPV) lasts seconds, migraine minutes, Meniere's disease hours and vestibular neuronitis days).
- Any triggering factors? (BPV, for example, is associated with head turning or patient adopting a certain head position).
- Any associated symptoms? (Vertigo of peripheral (vestibular) origin is commonly accompanied by nausea, vomiting, hearing disturbances and tinnitus).
- Any history or trauma or recent viral illness? (Head injury, for example, is associated with BPV; vestibular neuronitis may follow a recent viral illness).
- Past medical history (e.g. association between neurofibromatosis type 2 and acoustic neuroma; multiple sclerosis (MS) with brainstem demyelination causing vertigo of central origin).
- Current and past drug history (e.g. aminoglycosides (gentamicin) and streptomycin are vestibulotoxic drugs which may damage vestibular nerves resulting in persistent vertigo).

Differential diagnoses (Table 8.1)

Basic investigations
These will be guided by the results of history and detailed neurological examination, including a careful assessment of any nystagmus, cerebellar signs or gait abnormalities.
- Bedside hearing tests can be followed up with formal pure tone audiometry if indicated.
- Brainstem auditory evoked responses and calorimetry may be helpful.
- Investigations directed towards a possible central cause should include imaging (MRI of head—CT is a poor investigation for brainstem/cerebellar pathology) and possibly lumbar puncture (suspected MS).

Basic management
Refer to Table 8.1 on differential diagnoses.

Table 8.1 Clinical conditions causing vertigo with points to note

Clinical conditions	Points to note
Benign positional vertigo	Attacks of sudden onset of vertigo lasting seconds (<30 s) and precipitated by head turning. Due to displacement of otoconia in semicircular canal. Can follow head injury. Hallpike manoeuvre[a] may help in the diagnosis. *Treatment*: Self-limiting; physiotherapy (habituation); vestibular sedatives (prochlorperazine

(continued)

Table 8.1 (*Continued*)

Clinical conditions	Points to note
	or betahistine) may be used acutely but can maintain the problem over the medium/long term
Meniere's disease	Characterised by vertigo (lasting hours), nausea, vomiting, tinnitus and fluctuating sensorineural hearing loss. Attacks occur in clusters and are due to dilated endolymphatic spaces in membranous labyrinth. *Treatment*: Symptomatic for acute attacks with cyclizine and betahistine; further treatment may involve operative endolymphatic decompression (hearing conservation) or vestibular neurectomy (ipsilateral deafness)
Vestibular neuronitis	Severe vertigo with an abrupt onset and accompanied by nausea and vomiting. Vertigo lasts for days usually following a probable viral illness. Cyclizine for symptomatic treatment. Full recovery in 3–4 weeks
Central causes (MS, vertebrobasilar TIA, infarction and migraine)	Demyelination or infarction may lead to persistent vertigo compared to a TIA or migraine which produces more transient episodes. Hearing loss and tinnitus are less common in central causes. Nystagmus may be multidirectional, vertical and rotatory in central lesions compared to horizontal nystagmus in peripheral vestibular lesions. Look for associated cranial nerve signs to support a central cause
Acoustic neuroma	Schwannomma arising from superior vestibular division of the eighth nerve. Commonest cerebellopontine angle tumour. *Characteristic triad*: tinnitus, ipsilateral sensorineural hearing loss and disequilibrium or vertigo. *Treatment*: Surgical removal or stereotactic radiosurgery
Alcohol and vestibulotoxic drugs (aminoglycosides, for example gentamicin and streptomycin)	See above

[a]Hallpike manoeuvre involves (in a supine patient; head between examiner's hands) turning of patient's head to 30–40 degrees to one side and then rapid lowering of the head to 30 degrees below the level of the couch. In a peripheral cause, for example BPV, vertigo and nystagmus towards undermost ear after a latent period of 5–10 s are induced; this disappears within a minute or so and may reappear on sitting.

9   Weak legs

Weakness of the legs occurs due to various reasons:
- A few situations require emergent assessment followed by investigations and treatment, for example spinal cord compression due to an extradural metastatic tumour, cauda equina syndrome (CES) due to a herniated lumbar disc and Guillain–Barre syndrome (GBS).
- Follow detailed neurological history with an examination assessing tone (UMN versus LMN), pattern of weakness (unilateral versus bilateral), symmetric or asymmetric and proximal or distal, reflexes and plantar response (UMN versus LMN), evidence of sensory deficit and establishing a sensory level if present.

Remember: In cases of suspected CES, per-rectal examination is essential to document any loss of anal tone.

Useful selected questions to ask/facts to establish?
- Mode of onset and rate of progression (e.g. sudden onset implying a possible vascular (or ischaemic) aetiology versus gradual).
- Any evidence of weakness in upper limbs? (Useful for localisation as upper limb involvement points towards a lesion in cervical spine or brainstem or hemisphere; hemisphere lesions usually lead to contralateral weakness affecting face, arms and legs variably depending on the site of the lesion, whereas a cord lesion usually produces bilateral weakness with possible evidence of LMN signs at the level of the lesion and UMN signs below the level of the lesion with a sensory level).
- Presence of any associated pain with or without the history of malignancy? [(Pain is often the first symptom in patients with spinal extradural metastases (SEM) and can be radicular or referred, often worse with recumbency (at night) and with movement and can be bilateral in the thoracic region (radicular); presence of low back pain, bilateral sciatica, unilateral or bilateral weakness of dorsiflexion (foot drop) or plantarflexion may indicate the presence of CES; weakness may not be associated with any pain (e.g. in diabetes mellitus)].

Remember: Do not ignore bilateral radicular thoracic pain worse with recumbency in a patient, particularly with a known history of previous malignancy as they may have SEM requiring urgent attention. Common malignancies involving spine are lymphoma, lung, breast, prostate and those from GI tract.

- Any associated sensory loss (e.g. present in the setting of a cortical lesion, spinal cord lesion (look for a sensory level) and radiculopathy (involvement of nerve root) and in peripheral neuropathy; absent in diseases like motor neurone disease, neuromuscular junction problems, for example myasthenia gravis and primary muscle diseases).

Remember: Saddle anaesthesia (in the region of anus, perineum, lower genitals, buttocks and posterior superior thighs) is a common sensory abnormality associated with CES.

- Any evidence (from history or examination) of bowel and bladder involvement [e.g. urinary retention followed by overflow incontinence (preceded by hesitancy and other non-specific urinary complaints) is an important finding associated with CES; faecal

incontinence may also occur in CES; finally SEM compressing thoracic or cervical spine can also present with these symptoms including impotence].
- Evidence of spasticity versus flaccidity (spasticity with hyperreflexia implies an UMN lesion, therefore the lesion is in the spinal cord, brainstem or hemisphere; any lesion resulting in CES will cause a flaccid and areflexic weakness with this LMN pattern of weakness being seen in any peripheral cause from the anterior horn cell to the root, to the plexus and to the nerves).
- Establish whether patient is on anticoagulation therapy (e.g. warfarin leading to a spinal extradural haematoma with UMN signs).
- Any evidence of sepsis (raised inflammatory markers and temperature) with a recent history of staphylococcal infection suggests an extradural spinal abscess with associated back pain and tenderness on palpation.

Differential diagnoses (Table 9.1)

Basic investigations
- Guided by history and examination.
- *Blood tests*: FBC, U&E, calcium, ESR, B12, folate, LFT, PSA, syphilis and HIV serology and if suspected, serum electrophoresis for detecting multiple myeloma.
- Lumbar puncture (MS and GBS) in suspected cases.
- *Imaging*: MRI of spine (definitive investigation); CT of spine (fractures) usually preceded by plain X-ray of spine; chest X-ray, mammogram and CT chest, abdomen and pelvis if needed for detecting primary malignancy.

Basic management
- Guided by aetiology.
- *SEM-related cord compression*: High-dose steroids (dexamethasone), surgery (laminectomy), postoperative radiotherapy or radiotherapy alone without surgery.
- *CES*: Urgent discectomy if related to herniated lumbar disc.
- *Epidural abscess*: Appropriate antibiotics (initially intravenous followed by weeks of oral therapy) and surgery (laminectomy) if needed.

Table 9.1 Differential diagnoses for weak legs with points to note

Clinical presentations/ conditions	Points to note
Spastic paraparesis (Chapters 18 and 26)	Autoimmune conditions like MS, transverse myelitis; degenerative cervical or thoracic spinal stenosis; herniated intervertebral discs (cervical/thoracic); neoplastic process like extradural metastases, intradural extramedullary lesions, for example meningioma/neurofibroma, intradural intramedullary cord tumours, for example ependymoma and astrocytoma; subacute combined degeneration of the cord (SACD) due to vitamin B12 deficiency; infectious, for example spinal epidural abscess, tropical spastic paraparesis HTLV-1 infection; amyotrophic lateral sclerosis (ALS); spinal epidural haematoma (usually due to anticoagulation or trauma). *Note*: Trauma or cord infarction can cause spinal shock leading to acute cord syndrome presenting with flaccid weakness evolving to spastic paraparesis over days/weeks
Flaccid paraparesis (Chapter 24)	Peripheral neuropathies like Guillain–Barré syndrome and chronic inflammatory demyelinating polyneuropathy (CIDP) (diagnosed clinically and with nerve conduction studies); tabes dorsalis associated with

syphilis (occurs >15 years after infection due to damage to cauda equina and dorsal root ganglia); acquired muscle disease, for example polymyositis (normal sensation and initially persevered reflexes with raised creatine kinase)

SACD	Due to vitamin B12 deficiency (dietary or pernicious anaemia); subacute presentation with degeneration of dorsal column and corticospinal tracts; loss of joint position sense causing sensory ataxia and unsteadiness; progressive spasticity and paraplegia; visual disturbances with or without optic atrophy.

> *Remember: Can present with absent knee and ankle jerks with extensor plantars (also seen in ALS and Friederich's ataxia).*

Treatment is with B12 injections

Foot drop (Chapter 23)	Can be central (e.g. stroke) or peripheral. If peripheral, two possible sites need to be differentiated: (i) due to disc-related radiculopathy and (ii) due to common peroneal nerve palsy. L5 root compromise due to L4/L5 disc involves foot inversion which is spared if foot drop is due to a common peroneal nerve palsy. Also, history of back pain, sciatica and a characteristic distribution of sensory loss will favour L5 radiculopathy.

10   Numbness and sensory disturbance

Sensory disturbance is relatively common. Sensory symptoms are often non-specific and clarification is required via careful direct questioning. A full and detailed history, including drug history, is important for establishing the aetiology:
- 'Numbness' is described in various ways and may mean loss of sensation or heightened sensation or pain or even weakness. Paraesthesia (pins and needles/tingling) is usually described more accurately.
- Specifically ask about functional loss associated with sensory disturbance, for example clumsiness/unsteadiness with reduced proprioception (dorsal column) or inadvertent injury, for example burns, due to loss of pain and temperature sensation (spinothalamic tract).
- Performing a good sensory examination, due to its subjective nature, can be difficult and requires practice.

Useful selected questions to ask/facts to establish?
- Establish the character of the sensory disturbance (e.g. an absence of sensation (numbness), an uncomfortable sensation (dysaesthesia) or a burning or painful sensation).
- *Location*: Distribution of sensory symptoms and signs is important for anatomical localisation of the problem, i.e. brain, cord, root or roots, plexus, peripheral nerve or nerves. For example
  - Are the symptoms and signs in a specific dermatomal pattern implying a radiculopathy (nerve root entrapment) or in an area innervated by a single nerve (little and lateral half of ring finger in ulnar nerve entrapment)?
  - Is the problem more widespread and if so is this likely to be central or peripheral?
  - If central, is the problem in the brain where a contralateral hemisensory disturbance may be seen or in the cord where a bilateral sensory loss below the level of the lesion may occur?
  - If peripheral, are multiple nerves involved (polyneuropathy), and if so, are they large fibres (vibration and proprioceptive loss with loss of reflexes) or small fibres (burning pain) that are predominantly affected?

Remember: The characteristic glove and stocking (length dependent) distribution of peripheral neuropathy associated with diabetes.

- *Mode of onset and duration*: Establish whether sudden versus gradual and transient versus permanent? This helps in distinguishing between the different causes (e.g. transient disturbances in a migrainous episode, a focal seizure or a transient ischaemic attack; permanent sensory disturbance may imply a structural pathological lesion at different levels of the CNS and PNS, including a neoplasm or haematoma (subdural or intraparenchymal) or an infarct in the brain, spondylotic changes compressing the spinal cord and radiculopathy related to disc herniation in lumbar or cervical spine; demyelination, for example related to multiple sclerosis, may cause transient or permanent sensory disturbances).
- Associated disturbances (e.g. associated motor signs or sphincter (bowel and bladder) disturbances, specifically the presence of bowel and bladder dysfunction (e.g. urinary retention) in association with saddle anaesthesia (in the region of anus, perineum, genitals, and buttocks) and sciatica may raise the suspicion of cauda equina syndrome related to a herniated lumbar disc).

Remember: Sensory signs and symptoms should therefore always be put in the context of other associated deficits.

Differential diagnoses (Table 10.1)

Basic investigations

- Blood tests, including FBC, U&E, LFT (alcohol-related disease), fasting glucose levels (diabetes), and serum ACE (sarcoidosis).
- Nerve conduction studies (Chapter 4 for further details) to assess pattern and type of neuropathy if applicable (axonal versus demyelinating), somatosensory-evoked potentials and visual-evoked potentials (delayed in multiple sclerosis) and EEG (partial seizure).
- Imaging studies, including CT and MRI, of brain and spinal cord to assess for presence of structural lesions.

Basic management

This will depend upon the underlying cause. See relevant chapters in Part III.

Table 10.1 Clinical conditions leading to sensory disturbance with points to note

Clinical conditions	Points to note
Migraine (Chapter 12)	Short duration of onset (minutes) of unilateral sensory symptoms or aura, for example paraesthesia followed by other associated symptoms of migraine
Partial seizure (Chapter 17)	Unilateral onset over seconds of sensory disturbance, for example paraesthesia with or without the impairment of consciousness (simple versus complex partial seizure)
Transient ischaemic attack and stroke (Chapter 13)	Abrupt onset with or without other deficits. In stroke, there will be residual deficits beyond the 24 h period since onset
Structural lesions involving the parietal lobe (e.g. tumour, intracerebral haematoma) (Chapters 33, 34 and 36)	Contralateral neglect, agnosia, loss of position sense and two-point discrimination, inattention to a visual field
Radiculopathy (Chapter 23)	Can occur in cervical or lumbar spine as a result of herniated discs or trauma leading to compression of nerve roots. Associated with symptoms within the nerve root distribution
Peripheral neuropathy (Chapter 24)	Look for associated factors, for example systemic illness (diabetes, connective tissue diseases, and sarcoidosis), deficiency states (vitamins B1, B6, B12 and folate), drugs (amiodarone, cisplatinum, and isoniazid) and toxins (alcohol). Assess for other types of intrinsic peripheral neuropathy. Distribution and nerve conduction studies important for diagnosis
Non-organic	History of psychiatric illness, inconsistent and variable signs, normal investigations, including imaging studies

11   Gait assessment and disturbance

Gait assessment is an important part of the neurological examination:
- Gait disturbance may be due to dysfunction within the cortex, cerebral white matter tracts (including pyramidal or corticospinal tract), extrapyramidal system (basal ganglia), cerebellum, brainstem, spinal cord or peripheral nervous system.
- A peripheral gait disturbance may be due to abnormality within a single lumbosacral root or multiple roots, lumbosacral plexus, single or multiple peripheral nerves, the neuromuscular junction or skeletal muscle.
- Localisation of gait problem requires combining bed testing findings with gait observation.
- The aetiology, however, is often revealed by the temporal nature of the disturbance and by eliciting the presence or absence of particular associated features (e.g. a hyperacute onset of gait disturbance without associated pain or mechanical injury whether unilateral (brain) or bilateral (cord/brainstem) is likely to be vascular in origin, whereas a slowly progressive gait disturbance evolving over years is more likely to have a degenerative basis).

Useful selected questions to ask/facts to establish (during gait assessment)
- First, observe the patient attempting to arise from the chair or bed with their arms folded across their chest. Do they fall back into the chair and require more than one attempt? Do they require the use of their arms to push up or assistance to stand? Any staggering on arising? If struggling to stand, is there possible unilateral or bilateral lower limb disturbance?
- Posture on standing (e.g. stooped, normal or hypererect, position of the arms and head and neck).
- Ask the patient to walk forward for a minimum of 10 m, turn and walk back observing for and commenting upon gait initiation, stride length, cadence, corner turning, arm swing, gait base, unilateral weakness/dragging of a limb, waddling, foot drop, unsteadiness/veering or apparent discomfort/pain.
- Next ask them to close their eyes and perform a Romberg's test. A pull test assessing postural reflexes can also be performed (the examiner stands behind the patients and instructs them to maintain their balance when pulled backwards; the examiner pulls back briskly on the shoulders assessing the patient's ability to recover, being careful to prevent the patient from falling and noting whether they step back to save themselves or take several steps back before correcting or need to be caught).
- Depending on the clinical situation, further information is obtained by asking the patient to tandem walk, walk on their heels or on their toes or observe them running or walking backward.

Remember: It is important to ask about falls and if they have occurred, their frequency and the circumstances in which they have occurred.

Differential diagnoses

Clinical conditions (types of gait disturbance)	Points to note
Spastic hemiparesis/paraparesis	Due to brain, brainstem or cord disturbance, accompanied by upper motor neurone signs. The lower limb or limbs may be held in

	extension requiring circumduction of the limb on walking to avoid the front of the foot catching on the floor. Spontaneous clonus may be observed
Gait suggestive of extrapyramidal disorder (PD, MSA, PSP, CBD) (Chapter 19)	May take several attempts to stand, once stood posture is typically stooped with shortened stride length and steps, shuffling steps, festination, gait initiation failure, freezing, en bloc turning and absence of arm swing. Non-degenerative conditions may also produce short shuffling steps, gait initiation failure and freezing and include vascular parkinsonism, normal pressure hydrocephalus and drug-induced parkinsonism
Broad-based gait	May be due to a cerebellar or sensory ataxia. To distinguish, look for associated symptoms and signs of cerebellar dysfunction versus symptoms and signs associated with proprioceptive loss (positive Romberg's)
Foot drop (Chapters 9 and 23)	Can be central in origin, for example stroke or due to a peripheral disturbance, or seen in conditions with both upper and lower motor neuron signs, for example motor neurone disease
Waddling gait (Chapter 28)	Proximal lower limb weakness, which may be due to a disturbance of skeletal muscle leading to a waddling gait, problems in getting up from a chair and particular difficulty in getting up from a squatting position

Basic investigations
- Guided by the localisation of the problem and its likely aetiology.
- *MRI imaging*: An acute problem localising to the cervical or thoracic cord will require urgent MRI imaging of the cord at the clinically apparent level and above. MRI or CT brain is appropriate in a patient with a parkinsonian gait disorder possibly due to structural causes for example, normal pressure hydrocephalus.

Basic management
- Addressing the underlying cause. See relevant chapters in Part III (see differential diagnoses table above).
- Multidisciplinary approaches involving for example physiotherapy as well as appliances such as walking aids, ankle orthosis, and so on should be considered.
- Assessing and managing falls and falls risk is very important.

Part III
Conditions: Applying the basics

12   Headache

DEFINITION/DESCRIPTION   Headaches (also see Chapter 5) are a common reason for seeing the doctor and are considered to be either primary or secondary in origin. The commonest primary headache disorders are migraine, tension-type headache and cluster headache.

Migraine

The two commonest categories are migraine without aura and migraine with aura. A further category, often leading to a neurological referral, is chronic migraine. More than one category of migraine may occur in the same patient.

EPIDEMIOLOGY

- Very common and affects over 10% of people in the western world.
- *Prevalence*: Females (18%) > males (6%). It may commence at any age but most commonly the initial attack occurs during teens and a first episode of migraine is rare after the age of 40.
- Migraine beginning for the first time in older people requires investigation for alternative explanations.
- Tends to recur at variable frequency throughout life and attacks often become less severe and less frequent with age.

AETIOLOGY

- Approximately 90% have a family history.
- Modern neuroimaging techniques suggest a primary neural basis for migraine and pathophysiology may involve a neurovascular mechanism.

HISTORY

Migraine without aura: Diagnosis requires at least five lifetime attacks, lasting 4–72 h with two of four pain features and at least one of two sets of associated symptoms.

- *At least two of the following headache characteristics*: Unilateral new location, pulsating quality, moderate or severe pain intensity, aggravated or causing avoidance of routine physical activity (e.g. walking or climbing stairs).
- *At least one of the following associated features*: Nausea and/or vomiting, photophobia and/or phonophobia.

Migraine with aura: Typically migraine aura produces focal neurological symptoms which precede the headache but may occur without a following headache. Auras usually develop over 5 min and last no longer than an hour. Visual auras are by far the commonest. Sensory symptoms occur in approximately a third of patients with migraine with aura. Dysphasia and motor weakness, as well as decreased levels of consciousness may be seen but are far less common. The most frequent story in patients with migraine with aura is that the aura is followed by a headache with the features listed in the above section.

Remember: When attacks occur for 15 or more days per month, a diagnosis of chronic migraine can be made.

INVESTIGATIONS   A diagnosis of migraine is based on the history along with normal brain imaging. Patients should be reassured.

MANAGEMENT

- Reassurance regarding benign nature of migraine with no underlying sinister cause (such as a brain tumour) is important.

- *General recommendations*: Avoid triggers and reduce caffeinated drinks and alcohol intake, perform regular exercise with avoidance of prolonged fasts, have sufficient sleep and remove medications contributing to headaches.
- Pharmacotherapy can be divided into two groups. Therapies that provide symptomatic relief during an acute episode and therapies that are taken for their prophylactic effects if migraine frequency and duration are sufficient to warrant this. Typically, prophylactic regimens are considered if attacks occur more than several times each month.
- *Symptomatic treatment*: This is most effective if taken as early as possible during the attack. Simple analgesics such as Aspirin, Ibuprofen or Paracetamol may be all i.e. required with an antiemetic if necessary. If simple analgesics are not sufficient, *selective 5-HT1 agonists (Triptans)* may be used. Treat at least two different attacks before deciding a drug is ineffective. If there is no benefit from the drug, it may be necessary to change formulation or root of administration or add an adjunctive therapy. Non-drug treatments including lying in a darkened room or sleeping for a period are often effective towards shortening an attack.

> *Remember: Limit acute headache treatments to 2–3 times per week to minimise the risk of developing a medication overuse headache, which occurs secondary to frequent use of headache medications.*

- *Prophylactic treatment*: Relatively few preventative medications for migraine have proven to be effective in large randomised controlled clinical trials; therapies commonly tried in the United Kingdom include *Amitriptyline, Propranolol, Sodium Valproate and Topiramate*. Note that if the prophylactic drugs are used, administer it at a sufficient dose for a sufficient period of time (typically several months) before deeming them to be ineffective and moving to the next therapy.

Tension-type headache

Tension-type headache is the commonest primary headache disorder. Three sub-types are considered: infrequent episodic (where the headache episodes are less than 1 day per month), frequent episodic (where the episodes occur for 1–14 days per month) and chronic tension-type headache (where headaches occur for 15 or more days per month). In comparison to migraine-type headaches, these are relatively featureless.

HISTORY

- The main pain features are bilateral in location, non-pulsating quality, mild to moderate in intensity and lack of aggravation with routine physical activity.
- Not accompanied by nausea, though either photophobia or phonophobia may be present, and does not exclude the diagnosis.
- Chronic tension-type headaches typically evolve from episodic tension headaches. Episodic tension-type headaches last longer than 30 min and may continue for up to 7 days.

> *Remember: The major alternative differential of featureless tension-type headaches is medication overuse headaches.*

MANAGEMENT

- Reassurance of a non-sinister cause is often helpful in addition to techniques to promote relaxation of scalp and neck muscles. For infrequent mild tension-type headaches, Aspirin, Ibuprofen or Paracetamol may be sufficient. *Amitriptyline* is a helpful prophylactic agent. Chronic tension-type headaches may be chronic migraine and therefore if Amitriptyline fails, the alternative migraine prophylactic agents can be considered.

- Regular opioid use, and also simple analgesic overuse, should be particularly avoided due to the risk of developing a medication overuse headache.

Cluster headache

These are strictly unilateral and occur in association with cranial autonomic features. These are excruciatingly painful with attacks occurring in clusters and lasting weeks to months at a time. Episodes typically commence in the early hours of the morning.

EPIDEMIOLOGY
- The prevalence is approximately 0.1% and is much more common in men than in women. Typically presents in the third or fourth decade.

HISTORY
- Attacks have an abrupt start and finish; pain is located mainly round the orbital and temporal region and is strictly unilateral. Attacks usually last 45–90 min but can continue for up to several hours. Attacks commonly occur at the same time each night.
- A characteristic feature is the associated cranial autonomic symptoms, which last during the attack. In contrast to migraine patients (typically still during an episode), patients with cluster are often restless.

INVESTIGATIONS
- The diagnosis of cluster headaches is clinical. Secondary causes (due to a structural cause) exist and therefore an MRI scan of the brain is required.
- An alternative diagnosis is paroxysmal hemicranias, which is exquisitely sensitive to a specific treatment (Indomethacin) and therefore should be considered.

MANAGEMENT
- Patients are advised to abstain from alcohol during a cluster bout, as it may act as a trigger.
- *Subcutaneous Sumitriptan (5-HT1 agonist)*: It is useful during an acute episode. In relieving attacks, 100% oxygen is effective. A short course of Prednisolone may prevent attacks during a cluster bout. Relapse may occur at the end of a several weeks dosing period, therefore steroids are often used to control a cluster bout until longer acting prophylactic agents become effective.
- *Methysergide*: It can be used as a prophylactic agent but over the long term can cause fibrotic reactions. Long-term prevention may be achieved by the use of Verapamil.
- *Other therapy*: Injections of local anaesthetic and steroid around the greater occipital nerve on the affected side can abort a bout of cluster headache.

Brief notes on other conditions causing headache
Giant cell arteritis (GCA)

A condition characterised by chronic vasculitis (granulomatous arteritis) of large and medium-sized vessels (in particular affecting the external carotid artery). Usually seen in age >50 years (average age of onset around 70 years) with F:M = 2:1. Aetiology is unknown. Clinical symptoms include headache (commonest symptom), jaw claudication (pain on chewing) and visual disturbance, including amaurosis fugax and blindness, which is usually irreversible. Patients may also experience systemic symptoms, including fever and malaise, and may further have musculoskeletal symptoms ranging from aching and stiffness to weakness affecting proximal muscles like shoulders and hips (polymyalgia rheumatica). Examination in GCA may yield tenderness of temporal arteries (scalp tenderness) on palpation (alternatively patients may complain of pain on combing hair). ESR is usually elevated (>40 mm/h). Temporal artery biopsy is highly specific for the diagnosis. Treatment using high-dose steroids (e.g. prednisolone) eventually tapered gradually is aimed at relieving symptoms and preventing the irreversible complication of blindness.

Remember: Treatment with high-dose steroids in patients with a clinical suspicion of GCA should not be delayed in order to obtain a definitive diagnosis using temporal artery biopsy due to risk of blindness in this condition.

Idiopathic intracranial hypertension (IIH)

A condition characterised by increased intracranial pressure in the absence of a mass lesion or hydrocephalus. Also known as *pseudo-tumour cerebri or benign intracranial hypertension (Remember the condition is anything but benign!)*. It tends to affect obese women with a peak incidence in third decade. Associations include obesity, hypervitaminosis A, oral contraceptive use and others. Although by definition the condition is idiopathic, it may be secondary to venous sinus thrombosis. Symptoms classically include headache and visual disturbance, including transient blacking out of vision, constricted visual fields, poor colour vision and reduced visual acuity. Predominantly visual signs on examination are elicited and include papilloedema (extremely common), enlargement of blind spot with constricted visual fields and poor colour vision, reduced visual acuity and CN VI palsy (a false localising sign). CT or MRI with and without contrast is aimed at excluding both an intracranial mass lesion and a venous sinus thrombosis (using MR venography). Small slit-like ventricles may be seen. Lumbar puncture opening pressure in IIH patients is >20 cm H_2O with an otherwise normal cerebrospinal fluid analysis. All patients with suspected IIH should have a comprehensive opthalmological testing, including visual acuity, field testing (with perimetry), slit lamp examination and fundal photographs.

Remember: Spontaneous resolution may occur; however, these patients are at risk of permanent visual loss, so they require long-term follow-up and regular opthalmological evaluation.

Treatment options include weight loss and use of diuretics like *Acetazolamide (carbonic anhydrase inhibitor)*. If these fail, surgical options include optic nerve sheath fenestration (for those with visual loss without headache) or shunts (lumbo- or ventriculoperitoneal for patients with headache as the predominant feature of the disease).

Trigeminal neuralgia (TN)

TN is one of the craniofacial pain syndromes characterised by severe paroxysmal electric shock like pain, usually triggered by sensory stimuli including touching, shaving or eating and lasting a few seconds in the distribution of one or more divisions of the trigeminal nerve (i.e. ophthalmic—V1, maxillary—V2, mandibular—V3). It can be unilateral or bilateral (association with multiple sclerosis (MS). TN can occur in the context of neurovascular compression of the trigeminal nerve at its root entry zone (REZ) usually by a loop of superior cerebellar artery and other structural abnormalities like a posterior fossa tumour or in the context of demyelination in the brainstem, for example in MS. History is as above and examination is usually normal unless TN is associated with a tumour or is related to MS. MRI (with neurovascular protocol) is used to examine REZ for evidence of neurovascular compression, to look for other structural abnormalities like tumours or to exclude demyelinating plaques, for example in MS. Treatment is usually medical with use of drugs like Carbamazepine or Gabapentin. Surgical options (reserved for medically resistant cases or for cases with significant intolerable side effects from medications) include among others microvascular decompression via a retrosigmoid craniotomy (involving displacement of offending vessel from the REZ of trigeminal nerve) or percutaneous trigeminal rhizotomy (using glycerol injection or radio frequency coagulation). Spontaneous remission of TN may occur and last weeks to months.

13   Transient ischaemic attacks (TIAs)

DEFINITION   'An acute neurological event affecting cerebral or retinal function with symptoms lasting less than 24 hours.' This 24 h cut-off is arbitrary, and about one-third of patients with TIA fulfilling these criteria have evidence of ischaemic damage on brain MRI scanning. Therefore, a new definition was proposed by the American Stroke Association Stroke Council: 'A transient episode of neurological dysfunction caused by focal brain, spinal cord, or retinal ischemia, without acute infarction.'

EPIDEMIOLOGY
- *Incidence* : ↑ *with age*: Estimates vary widely and TIAs are probably still underrecognised.
- *The general incidence in the United Kingdom*: Around 0.5 per 1000 in the population as a whole, rising to an estimated 6.4 per 1000 in people over 85 years (data from OXVASC population study, Oxford, UK, 2002–2004).

AETIOLOGY AND PREVENTION   Aetiology similar to thromboembolic stroke (see Chapter 14) and due to an artery-to-artery emboli or cardiac emboli. Prevention includes management of risk factors, i.e. antihypertensives (not beta-blockers), good diabetic control, cholesterol-lowering agents, regular exercise, smoking cessation, limitation of alcohol intake (particularly binge drinking) and judicious use of HRT in high-risk patients.

ASSOCIATIONS/RISK FACTORS
- *Principal risk factors*: Atrial fibrillation (AF), hypertension, current smoking, diabetes, hypercholesterolaemia and family history. Other vascular disease (ischaemic heart disease and peripheral vascular disease), prior TIA or stroke.
- *Other risk factors/associations*: Excess alcohol (binge drinking), polycythaemia, drugs, for example combined OCP and HRT, race, obesity and physical inactivity, raised CRP and plasma homocysteine, and lower socio-economic status.

CLINICAL FEATURES (HISTORY/EXAMINATION)
Clinicians, including stroke specialist neurologists, often disagree about perceived likelihood of a TIA diagnosis.
- *Clinical features making diagnosis of TIA*: More likely include rapid onset (within seconds), history suggestive of typical vascular syndrome, especially carotid territory (see Chapter 14) and physical signs corresponding to symptoms and multiple risk factors for TIA.
- *Features decreasing likelihood for TIA*: Previous unexplained neurological symptoms and non-specific symptoms such as dizziness without vertigo, syncope and cognitive impairment.
- *Amaurosis fugax*: Type of TIA characterized by sudden loss of monocular vision, either complete (central retinal artery) or sectoral/central (branch retinal artery). The central retinal artery originates from the ophthalmic artery, a branch of the internal carotid artery.

INVESTIGATIONS
- *Brain imaging*: Useful to differentiate between TIA and mimics and exclude intracranial haemorrhage (CT) and to identify patients with cerebral infarction (diffusion-weighted MRI).
- *Arterial imaging*:
  - *Carotid Doppler ultrasound*: Detects narrowing using blood flow velocity and may identify plaque features reflecting risk. Limited by calcification and arterial anatomy.
  - *CT angiography (CTA) and contrast MR angiography* (MRA): More accurate than carotid Doppler ultrasound, and can evaluate *intracranial* arterial stenosis. Beware that contrast agents carry risks for patients with renal impairment.
- *Electrocardiography (ECG)*: Arrhythmias (particularly AF) and myocardial infarction (may indicate ventricular aneurysm)

- *Echocardiography*: Valvular heart disease, for example mitral valve disease (association with AF), enlarged left atrium (also associated with atrial fibrillation) and intracardiac thrombus. Use of a contrast agent (micro-bubbles) may show a patent foramen ovale.
- *Cardiac rhythm monitoring*: Asymptomatic AF may be detected using cardiac rhythm monitoring, for example ward-based monitoring or 24 h tape.

MANAGEMENT

Early assessment: The risk of stroke is highest very early after TIA; therefore, patients with suspected TIA require easy and rapid access to specialist review and investigation. For moderate and high-risk patients (e.g. ABCD2 score of 4 or above), this is typically within 24 h. For low-risk patients, it may be reasonable for review to occur within 7 days.

Medical management (see Chapter 14): According to two studies (SOS-TIA and EXPRESS), medical management alone can reduce 30 day stroke risk by 80% following TIA. Patients with AF (including paroxysmal AF) have a significant risk of stroke after TIA of about 4–18% per annum, depending on the presence of other risk factors such as age, hypertension, congestive cardiac failure and diabetes.

> *Remember the association between AF and the risk of TIA/stroke.*

- *Antiplatelet agents*: With proven benefit include Aspirin, dipyridamole (*Modified release* dipyridamole reduces risk of stroke following TIA, over and above *only in combination with aspirin*. Immediate release preparations appear to be *ineffective*) and clopidogrel.
  - *Initial treatment*: Aspirin 300 mg daily, aspirin 75 mg + dipyridamole modified release 200 mg bd or clopidogrel 75 mg daily are reasonable. In high-risk patients, a combination of aspirin 75 mg and clopidogrel 75 mg daily, after loading with 300 mg of each drug, may be beneficial.
  - *Subsequent treatment (e.g. after 14 days)*: A combination of aspirin and modified release dipyridamole is more effective than aspirin alone (ESPRIT and ESPS2 trials). Clopidogrel appears to be equivalent to aspirin and dipyridamole in combination (PROFESS trial).
- *Anticoagulants*: Patients with AF should be started on anticoagulants after TIA as soon as haemorrhage is excluded by brain imaging (with CT). Warfarin is currently the most effective drug for prevention of stroke after TIA in AF (WARRS trial versus aspirin, ACTIVE-W trial versus aspirin/clopidogrel combination), but causes more haemorrhagic strokes. Aspirin 75–100 mg daily plus clopidogrel 75 mg daily prevents more strokes than aspirin alone, but causes more haemorrhages of all types (ACTIVE-A trial). Clopidogrel is not currently licensed in the United Kingdom for treatment of TIA, but in combination with aspirin this is a reasonable alternative to warfarin in patients unable to take warfarin, for example due to high risk of falls.

> *Remember: Warfarin is the most effective drug for prevention of stroke after TIA in AF.*

Dabigatran is a new anticoagulant, at least as effective as warfarin in preventing stroke in atrial fibrillation, with equal or lower haemorrhage rates (RELY study).
- *Antihypertensive agents*: The strongest evidence for prevention of stroke (PROGRESS trial, *Lancet* 2001) is for a combination of a thiazide diuretic (specifically indapamide) and an ACE inhibitor (specifically perindopril). Beta-blockers appear to be relatively *ineffective* in preventing stroke.
- *Cholesterol-lowering agents*: Statins significantly reduce the risk of stroke in patients with cerebrovascular disease and cholesterol levels of ≥ 3.6. Simvastatin 40 mg once daily is a suitable initial treatment.

Surgical management: Carotid endarterectomy and stenting:
- Endarterectomy reduces death and stroke in patients with carotid stenosis of $\geq$70% (loss of $\geq$70% of the lumen) on the side corresponding to symptoms.
- *Endarterectomy benefits patients with 50–69% stenosis if performed*: On patients with low surgical risk and by surgeons with low complication rates.
- *Endarterectomy*: Perform as soon as possible after the index event, provided the patient is stable (usually within 2 weeks). Lower rate of immediate complications (especially non-disabling stroke) than endovascular stenting and has greatest benefit over stenting in older patients. Stenting is equivalent to endarterectomy in young patients. Use aspirin both before and following endarterectomy to reduce embolic complications.

Lifestyle modifications: Following TIA, these are important: smoking cessation, improved diabetic control (including medication, exercise and low glycaemic index diet), dietary changes (especially low saturated fat and low salt), increased exercise (5 or more days per week, 30 or more min duration each to slight breathlessness), weight loss in obese patients, alcohol reduction to recommended limits (3 units per day for men, 2 units for women per day in the United Kingdom) with avoidance of binge drinking and avoidance of the combined oral contraceptive and HRT.

PROGNOSIS   Although TIAs by definition completely resolve, they are often markers of significant risk.
- About 15% of strokes are preceded by a TIA, and within a year of TIA up to a quarter of patients die.
- About half of the patients going on to have a stroke within 30 days after TIA have their stroke within 24 h.
- *Factors associated with increased risk of stroke after TIA*: Carotid stenosis, abnormality on diffusion-weighted MRI (early after TIA this may show ischaemic changes which approximate to areas of acute infarction), repeated TIA events over a short period (e.g. 1 month or less), increasing age, hypertension, clinical features—hemiparesis and speech disturbance, symptom duration and diabetes.
- Patients must be advised to inform the Driver and Vehicle Licensing Agency (DVLA) of being advised to not to drive for 1 month following a TIA (due to risk of further TIA and stroke). If there are no symptoms after this time, patients may start driving again.
- *Individualising risk of stroke after TIA*: The ABCD2 score (Table 13.1) is widely used to estimate individual risk of stroke after TIA and guide management. Patients are scored (total score range 0–7) and then categorised as low, medium or high risk.

Table 13.1 ABCD2 score to estimate individual risk of stroke after TIA

Calculation of ABCD2 score		Estimation of individual stroke risk				
Risk factor	Add score	Total score	Risk stratum	% Risk of stroke within time		
				2 days	7 days	90 days
Age 60 years or more	1	0–3	Low	1.0	1.2	3.1
First BP $\geq$ 140/90	1	4–5	Moderate	4.1	5.9	9.8
Clinical features		6–7	High	8.1	11.7	17.8
Speech disturbance	1					

(continued)

Table 13.1 (*Continued*)

Calculation of ABCD2 score		Estimation of individual stroke risk				
Risk factor	Add score	Total score	Risk stratum	% Risk of stroke within time		
				2 days	7 days	90 days
Unilateral weakness	2					
Duration						
10–59 min	1					
60 min or more	2					
Diabetes	1					

DIFFERENTIAL DIAGNOSES (TABLE 13.2)

Table 13.2 Differential diagnoses for TIA with points to note

Clinical conditions	Points to note
Hypoglycaemia	Check blood glucose (usually capillary) immediately in all patients with suspected stroke or TIA
Migraine (Chapter 12)	Migraine aura resulting from temporary cerebral dysfunction can be mistaken for TIA. History and sequence of events important
Seizures (Chapter 17)	Todd's paresis following a seizure, and focal seizures may cause symptoms mimicking TIA. Stereotyped symptoms typically suggest seizures
Syncope (Chapter 6)	Loss of consciousness/blackouts is uncommon in TIA but can occur in posterior circulation TIAs with abrupt onset without prodrome. Accompanying brainstem symptoms are helpful in discriminating TIA from syncope
Previous stroke with intercurrent illness	Patients with cerebral damage from previous stroke frequently have recurrence of their stroke symptoms when systemically unwell, for example due to infection
Vestibular disorders	Can cause vertigo of abrupt onset mimicking vertebrobasilar TIA
Functional symptoms	Deficit (e.g. hemiparesis) without organic illness is uncommon
Pressure palsies (radial nerve palsy)	Differentiate using history from TIA

14   Stroke I: Thromboembolic stroke and syndromes

DEFINITION   A stroke is a neurological deficit (usually focal but sometimes global) of cerebrovascular cause that persists beyond 24 h or leads to death within 24 h.

EPIDEMIOLOGY   Stroke is the third largest cause of death and the largest cause of severe disability in the United Kingdom and the United States. Around 150 000 people have a stroke each year in the United Kingdom; at any one time, over 300 000 people have moderate to severe disability because of stroke. Age-specific incidence of first-ever stroke in the United Kingdom is shown in Table 14.1. More than three-quarters of first-ever strokes occur in over 65 s. Approximately 90% of all strokes are ischaemic in origin (rather than haemorrhagic).

Stroke incidence is higher in males at young ages and in females at older ages. The incidence of stroke in the United Kingdom is falling.

AETIOLOGY   The commonest causes of thromboembolic stroke, particularly in older patients, are as follows:
- Large-artery atherosclerosis (internal carotid, vertebral, basilar, aorta and middle cerebral arteries).
- Cardioembolism, for example from atrial fibrillation, and left ventricular aneurysm.
- Small-vessel occlusion, causing lacunar stroke (see Section 'Clinical Syndromes').
- Arterial dissection with embolism, especially internal carotid artery (look for Horner's syndrome), and vertebral arteries (a common cause of stroke in young patients, for example following minor neck trauma, and probably underrecognised in older patients, in whom one of the above causes may be presumed).

Among the less common causes of stroke (mostly young onset) are the following:
- Patent foramen ovale (PFO) with paradoxical embolism from venous thrombosis.
- Antiphospholipid syndrome.
- Vasculitis (usually young onset except giant cell arteritis).

Table 14.1 Total incidence of stroke (males and females) in the OXVASC study, Oxford, UK

Age (years)	Incidence per 1000 population
<35	0
35–44	0.2
45–54	0.6
55–64	1.8
65–74	5.3
75–84	10.1
85+	16.5

- CADASIL (cerebral autosomal dominant arteriopathy with subcortical infarcts and leukoencephalopathy).
- Fabry disease (alpha-galactosidase A deficiency) (rare).
- Mitochondrial disorder (MELAS) (rare).
- Homocystinuria (rare).

ASSOCIATIONS/RISK FACTORS
- Principal risk factors are the same as for transient ischaemic attack (see Chapter 13).
- *Racial differences in incidence and risk factors*: Stroke is approximately one-fifth more common in males of African, Caribbean, and South Asian origin than in white males, and one-third more common in females. Hypertension and diabetes are also more common in these ethnic groups.

Clinical syndromes

HISTORY/EXAMINATION   Because of the anatomy of the cerebral vasculature, thromboembolic stroke tends to result in particular sets of symptoms and signs or 'stroke syndromes'. Many of these are uncommon or rare (examples can be reviewed at the Internet Stroke Center www.strokecenter.org/prof/syndromes/). For more common stroke types, the OCSP classified strokes into broad syndromes to aid prediction of prognosis. Though more than 20 years old, these syndromes are still useful; they are described below. Anterior circulation refers to the territory of an internal carotid artery—middle cerebral artery and/or anterior cerebral artery. Posterior circulation refers to the territory of the vertebral and basilar arteries.
- *Total anterior circulation stroke (TACS)*: Results from occlusion of the internal carotid artery or proximal middle cerebral artery:
  - Contralateral hemiparesis with or without sensory deficit involving two or more out of three body areas (face/upper limb/lower limb) opposite the lesion.
  - Homonymous visual field defect opposite the lesion.
  - Higher cortical dysfunction (dysphasia, neglect, visuospatial problems, depending on the hemisphere affected and cerebral dominance).
- *Partial anterior circulation stroke (PACS)*: Results from occlusion of a branch of the middle cerebral artery. The PACI syndrome reflects less extensive neuronal loss than the TACI syndrome, comprising two of the three deficits listed above or as follows:
  - Isolated higher cortical dysfunction (i.e. isolated dysphasia or predominantly proprioceptive deficit in one limb), *or*
  - Motor/sensory deficits restricted to *one part of the body* (face/arm/leg contralateral to the lesion).
- *Posterior circulation stroke (POCS)*:
  - Isolated (or occasionally bilateral) homonymous haemianopia due to occipital cortex damage.
  - Brainstem ischaemia with cranial nerve involvement ipsilateral to the lesion (diplopia, vertigo, dysphonia and dysarthria) and/or various patterns of ophthalmoplegia, as well as ipsilateral long-tract motor signs and contralateral sensory signs (e.g. the lateral medullary syndrome or Wallenberg syndrome).
  - Cerebellar ischaemia with ipsilateral limb (cerebellar hemispheres) and trunk (midline cerebellum) ataxia, vomiting, vertigo with horizontal nystagmus, and usually mild ipsilateral limb weakness.
  - Midbrain ischaemia with a variety of possible signs of both anterior and posterior circulation syndromes, with or without somnolence or behavioural disturbance.
- *Lacunar stroke (LACS)*: Results from *in situ* thrombosis of small end arteries to basal ganglia and internal capsule or of small arteries in the 'watershed zones' between vascular territories. Hypertensive, diabetic patients are particularly at risk.

Lacunar strokes are small lesions, usually deep within the brain. They typically do not cause visual field defects, cortical deficits, depression of consciousness or brainstem signs. The three commonest lacunar syndromes are as follows:

o *Pure motor*: A unilateral motor deficit (internal capsule or pons).
o *Pure sensory*: Similar to motor in distribution, proprioception is spared (thalamus).
o *Sensorimotor*: Combined deficit (thalamus and internal capsule).

Many others exist, for example ataxic hemiparesis, dysarthria clumsy hand syndrome.

INVESTIGATIONS   See Chapter 13.

MANAGEMENT   Treatment follows the following principles:
- *Restoration of blood flow*: Usually thrombolysis, possible only in some carefully selected patients.
- *Prevention and treatment of complications*: For example aspiration pneumonia, thromboembolism, spasticity, depression and seizures.
- *Rehabilitation*: Physical, occupational, vocational, speech therapy and neuropsychological rehabilitation.
- *Secondary prevention*: For example antiplatelet and anticoagulant therapy, treatment of hypercholesterolaemia and treatment of hypertension.
- *Long-term support*: (beyond the scope of this chapter).

Stroke units
Stroke units should be the place of care for stroke patients. Staffed with multidisciplinary stroke specialists, they reduce the relative risk of patient death by about 15% and institutional care by about 20%. A stroke unit is more effective than either a stroke bay on a medical ward or a mobile stroke team.

Thrombolysis
The clot dissolving drug recombinant tissue plasminogen activator (rt-PA), and possibly others (though not streptokinase), has been shown to improve outcome in ischaemic stroke in carefully selected patients. Unfortunately, the majority of patients are not eligible for treatment, either because they attend hospital too long after the onset of symptoms or because they have another contraindication to treatment.

The following are the important facts related to recombinant tissue plasminogen activator given intravenously within $3–4\frac{1}{2}$ h:
- Is more effective the earlier it is given.
- Reduces frequency of death or dependency at around 6 months by about one-third (relative risk) on average.
- Increases early death due to intracranial haemorrhage by approximately three–four times.
- Is more likely to cause haemorrhage the later it is given.
    Did not affect overall mortality at the end of patient follow-up in clinical trials.

Alternatives to intravenous thrombolysis include the following:
- *Intra-arterial thrombolysis*: This appears to be effective up to 6 h after the onset of symptoms.
- *Intra-arterial clot extraction*: This appears to be the most effective method for restoring blood flow, but its effectiveness has not been proven in terms of clinical outcomes. Unlike intravenous thrombolysis, it can be attempted in patients taking oral anticoagulation.
- *Combinations of intravenous thrombolysis and the above treatments*.

Aspirin
A dose of 300 mg of aspirin daily given as soon as possible after stroke for 14 days improves outcomes at 6 months and reduces recurrent ischaemic strokes within 14 days (absolute risk reduction 1.1% and relative risk reduction 28% in the International Stroke Trial).

MEDICAL MANAGEMENT: SECONDARY PREVENTION   Standard medical management for secondary prevention of thromboembolic stroke in patients without atrial fibrillation is as follows:

- Rule out intracerebral haemorrhage, for example with brain CT.
- Aspirin 300 mg od immediately (clopidogrel 75 mg od if aspirin intolerant).
- Change to combination of aspirin 75 mg od + dipyridamole MR 200 mg bd after perhaps 2 weeks (clopidogrel 75 mg od alone if either drug not tolerated).

For all patients with thromboembolic stroke:

- If cholesterol is ≥3.6, start simvastatin 40 mg nocte (MRC Heart Protection Study). Other agents, for example fibrates, may be used in patients unable to tolerate statins. Because of the potential risk of haemorrhage associated with statin use, NICE does not recommend immediate statin use (e.g. wait 72 h from stroke before starting statins).
- If systolic BP is ≥110 mmHg, start antihypertensives, aiming for treatment with an ACE inhibitor and a thiazide diuretic (best evidence is the PROGRESS trial, in which perindopril 4 mg daily plus indapamide 2.5 mg daily reduced relative stroke risk by 43% compared to placebo). The role of acute blood pressure lowering after stroke remains unclear.

Further antiplatelet options:

- As suggested by the EXPRESS trial, in patients with minor stroke without atrial fibrillation in whom treatment can be started within 48 h (i.e. within the highest risk period), it may be reasonable to give aspirin 75 mg plus clopidogrel 75 mg (after a 300 mg loading dose of aspirin) for a month, followed by aspirin 75 mg plus dipyridamole MR 200 mg bd.

Further cholesterol-lowering treatment:

- Treatment should be increased for patients who fail to reach a target of 4 mmol/L total cholesterol or 2 mmol/L LDL cholesterol (NICE guideline). High doses of statins (atorvastatin 80 mg) may increase the rate of intracerebral haemorrhage following stroke (SPARCL study).
- Further antihypertensives.
- Treatment should be further increased if a target blood pressure of 140 mmHg systolic and 90 mmHg diastolic is not met (NICE guideline).

Atrial fibrillation:

- Patients with atrial fibrillation should be considered for anticoagulation. In patients with stroke, there is an increased risk of intra-cerebral haemorrhage with all anticoagulants, therefore a period (usually 2 weeks) should be left between the stroke and starting anticoagulant medication. For further principles of anticoagulant management in atrial fibrillation, see Chapter 2.

Nutrition and feeding Dysphagia with aspiration is common in stroke, though dysphagia usually resolves in surviving patients. The FOOD series of clinical trials found the following:

- Early nasogastric feeding appears to improve survival, but this may be at the expense of increased dependent survival.
- Percutaneous endoscopic gastrostomy (PEG) should be reserved for patients in whom nasogastric feeding cannot be used or who require prolonged feeding.
- *Routine* nutritional supplementation does not improve outcomes.

Thromboprophylaxis Deep venous thrombosis with or without pulmonary embolism is common following stroke, particularly in hemiplegic and non-ambulant patients. All anticoagulants increase the risk of haemorrhage following stroke; in the acute phase, this generally exceeds any benefit. However, thromboprophylaxis with low-molecular weight heparin may be beneficial after the acute period, in patients with low risk of bleeding (e.g. no haemorrhagic transformation of the cerebral infarct) and high risk of thromboembolism. (e.g. severe immobility/hemiplegia, dehydration, previous venous thromboembolism and comorbidity such as cancer).

Carotid endarterectomy and stenting Carotid endarterectomy may be indicated for patients following a stroke if they have shown a reasonable recovery (reflecting a reasonable capacity to benefit from the procedure). For further details, see Chapter 13.

COMPLICATIONS   Complications after stroke include the following:

- *Aspiration pneumonia*: Dysphagia after stroke puts patients at risk of aspiration and therefore pneumonia.
- *Venous thromboembolism*: Deep venous thrombosis (DVT) is common after stroke, and pulmonary embolism (PE) is not infrequent. Severe weakness and immobility put patients at high risk. The CLOTS trial showed no benefit of thigh-length compression stockings in stroke patients. Anticoagulants used to prevent and treat DVT and PE can cause bleeding into damaged brain, therefore their use often involves a difficult risk/benefit assessment (see above).
- *Depression*: Depression is common after stroke. Antidepressants can be beneficial. Psychological therapies may also have benefit.
- *Spasticity*: Spasticity, or increased muscle tone, after stroke can be painful and interfere with function. Physiotherapy, antispasmodic medication, such as baclofen, and botulinum toxin are the main treatments. Intrathecal baclofen and surgery for contractures are less commonly used.
- *Seizures*: Seizures may occur early (within 2 weeks, about half within 24 h) or late (after 2 weeks) after stroke. Late seizures have a higher rate of recurrence; about one-third of patients with early seizures and one-half with late seizures go on to epilepsy.

Note on rehabilitation

Rehabilitation should begin soon after stroke, though it is not clear exactly how early this should happen. Physiotherapy improves gait and aims to restore other aspects of physical function, while reducing risk of falls. Occupational therapy aims to improve function by, for example, simplifying and practising tasks. Speech and language therapy aims to improve speech production, intelligibility and comprehension and swallowing ability. Speech and language therapists regularly assess aspiration risk to guide decisions about route of feeding. Rehabilitation goals should be set and their attainment regularly reviewed. More detailed discussion of stroke rehabilitation is beyond the scope of this chapter.

PROGNOSIS   The natural history of the major subtypes of thromboembolic stroke was investigated on a population scale in the Oxford Community Stroke Project (1981–1984). Table 14.2 shows prognosis at 1 year in terms of outcome and recurrent stroke.

Table 14.2 Natural history of stroke at 1 year (data from the Oxford Community Stroke Project)

	LACI (%)	TACI (%)	PACI (%)	POCI (%)	All patients
Dead	11	60	16	19	23
Dependent	28	36	29	19	28
Independent	60	4	55	62	49
Recurrent stroke	9	6	17	20	14

DIFFERENTIAL DIAGNOSES (ALSO SEE TABLE 13.2) The differential diagnosis of thromboembolic stroke is similar to that of TIA, though there are differences (Table 14.3).

Table 14.3 Differential diagnoses for thromboembolic stroke with points to note

Clinical conditions	Points to note
Subdural haematoma (Chapter 33)	This is not conventionally classed as a stroke. Brain scans should be examined closely as small subdural haematomas are easily missed
Subarachnoid haemorrhage (Chapter 16)	Subarachnoid haemorrhage is sometimes classified as a type of stroke. Along with the typical sudden onset of severe headache, it can cause focal neurological deficits
Migraine (Chapter 12)	Migraine aura results from temporary cerebral dysfunction. It generally does not last more than 24 h but sometimes can. Migraine with aura may itself occasionally cause stroke
Previous stroke with intercurrent illness	Patients with cerebral damage from previous stroke frequently have recurrence of their stroke symptoms when they are systemically unwell, for example due to infection
Epileptic seizure (Chapter 17)	Though Todd's paresis (weakness persisting after a seizure) does not generally last 24 h, in patients with ongoing recurrent focal seizures or in patients with severe generalised seizures and previous focal brain damage, seizures may mimic stroke
Functional symptoms	Symptoms, especially hemiparesis, in the absence of organic illness are surprisingly common. The duration of symptoms is variable
Vestibular disorders (Chapter 8)	Vestibular disease can cause vertigo of abrupt onset and mimic vertebrobasilar stroke
Pressure palsies, for example radial nerve palsy	These can usually be differentiated in the history but can cause difficulty in patients with multiple vascular risk factors, particularly as acute stroke often presents with flaccid tone
Hypoglycaemia	Hypoglycaemia can precipitate stroke but will not usually cause symptoms for more than 24 h duration

15 Stroke II: Intracerebral haemorrhage

DEFINITION   Intracerebral haemorrhage (ICH) refers to haemorrhage within the parenchyma of the brain.

EPIDEMIOLOGY   Approximately 15 cases/100 000 per year. ICH accounts for 15–30% of all strokes (second commonest form of stroke after thromboembolic CVAs).

AETIOLOGY
- *Hypertension*: Chronic hypertension implicated as a major risk factor for spontaneous ICH. Hypertension due to eclampsia or preeclampsia may also present with ICH.
- *Underlying vascular abnormality*: Arteriovenous malformations (AVMs)—younger patients (≤45 years) with lobar haemorrhages, cerebral aneurysms (see Chapter 16) and cavernoma (low-volume haemorrhage and evidence of previous bleeding).
- *Coagulation disorders*: These may be iatrogenic as a consequence of anticoagulation/antiplatelet therapy, particularly in subgroup of patients with poorly regulated INR on warfarin or in patients receiving thrombolysis (alteplase) for either an ischaemic stroke or myocardial infarction. Thrombocytopenia or coagulopathy related to any other cause including medications or liver dysfunction.
- *Cerebral amyloid angiopathy (CAA)*: Common cause of ICH in the elderly presenting with recurrent lobar/cortical haemorrhages with underlying pathology involving deposition of beta amyloid in media of small cortical vessels.
- *Brain tumours*: Those likely to haemorrhage include metastatic lesions (melanoma, choriocarcinoma and renal cell carcinoma) and glioblastoma multiforme (GBM).
- *Trauma*: Including haemorrhagic contusion.
- *Infection*: Related to mycotic aneurysms and infectious vasculitis.
- Recreational drug abuse (cocaine and amphetamine: sympathomimetic agents) and chronic alcohol abuse.
- Venous sinus thrombosis.

ASSOCIATIONS/RISK FACTORS   In addition to the above, risk factors for spontaneous ICH: sex (M > F), increasing age (above 50–55 years of age), race (more common in African-Americans) and alcohol and drug abuse. Include questions specifically directed towards ascertaining the presence of any of the aetiological factors as above.

PATHOLOGY/PATHOGENESIS   Spontaneous ICH usually occurs secondary to rupture of small penetrating vessels into brain parenchyma in basal ganglia, thalamus, pons or cerebellum, related to small vessel disease due to hypertension. Chronic hypertension causes degenerative changes within blood vessels and formation of microaneurysms of Charcot–Bouchard, occurring principally at bifurcation points of small perforating branches of lenticulostriate arteries (branch of middle cerebral artery) in basal ganglia. Clinical signs and subsequent deterioration is related to direct injury to brain from haemorrhage and further damage due to mass effect, hydrocephalus and increased intracranial pressure.

HISTORY   Symptoms of raised intracranial pressure (see Chapter 30) with a focal neurological deficit (see below).

EXAMINATION   Focal neurological deficits associated with spontaneous ICH may have a progressive onset, usually over minutes, unlike thromboembolic episodes which have a maximal deficit at the onset. Common sites are deep structures, including basal ganglia (50%) and thalamus (15%), pons (10%), cerebellum (10%) and cerebral hemispheres (lobar) (10–20%). Haemorrhage in the putamen, thalamus, pons and cerebellum are typically linked to hypertension. Clinical findings based on location are as follows:
- *Putaminal*: Commonest site for ICH, causes contralateral hemiparesis or hemiplegia with conjugate deviation of the eyes ipsilateral to the side of the haematoma.

- *Thalamic*: Classically characterised by contralateral hemisensory loss or changes with dominant thalamic involvement also causing dysphasia. Small unreactive pupils with vertical gaze palsy with midbrain involvement.
- *Cerebellar*: Can rapidly lead to clinical deterioration and coma as a result of direct brainstem compression or hydrocephalus from either the compression or the extension of haemorrhage into the fourth ventricle. Signs of cerebellar dysfunction (see Chapter 3).
- *Pontine*: Coma with pinpoint unreactive pupils, quadriparesis or quadriplegia and respiratory disturbances, often fatal.
- Lobar (see Chapter 3 for lobar syndromes).

INVESTIGATIONS

- *Routine blood tests*: FBC (including platelet count), U & E (check for evidence of end organ damage related to hypertension and hyponatraemia related to SIADH), LFT, G & S, clotting profile (PT, APTT, and INR).
- *ECG*: Look for evidence of left ventricular hypertrophy.
- *Imaging*:
  - *CT*: Initial diagnostic investigation of choice, can be done rapidly and shows blood as high density (brighter) compared to brain parenchyma immediately after the event, shows degree of midline shift and mass effect, presence of associated intraventricular extension with or without hydrocephalus (Figure 15.1).
  - *MRI*: Useful at a delayed interval for demonstrating underlying structural abnormalities, for example a tumour.

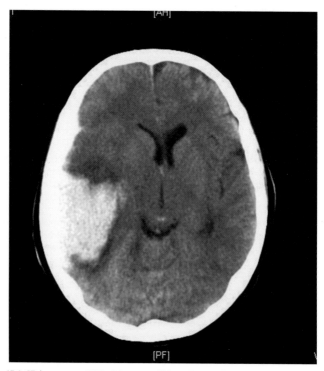

Figure 15.1 CT demonstrates ICH in right temporal lobe with mass effect and effacement of ipsilateral frontal horn of right lateral ventricle.

- o *Cerebral angiography*: Generally recommended unless patients are above 45 years of age with known hypertension and have haemorrhage in putamen or thalamus. An angiogram should not delay the initial emergency treatment if required and can be performed at a delayed interval to increase the diagnostic yield.

Remember: CT head is the initial diagnostic investigation of choice in ICH.

MANAGEMENT
Non-surgical

Remember that adequate attention to airways and breathing and circulation (ABC) and securing of airway is particularly required in patients with low GCS ($\leq$8).

- *Hypertension*: Slowly reduce blood pressure to patients' premorbid levels if known; if not, aim for a 20% reduction in BP. Too rapid a correction, particularly in the presence of raised intracranial pressure, could lead to hypoperfusion and infarction. In initial stages, most patients with ICH will present with high BP irrespective of presence of premorbid hypertension due to increased ICP.
- Correct any coagulopathy and stop any anticoagulant or antiplatelet medications. The following agents may be considered: fresh frozen plasma (coagulopathy), vitamin K and prothrombin complex concentrate (PCC) for warfarin; protamine sulphate for unfractionated heparin; platelet transfusion for patients with thrombocytopenia (<50 000) or taking aspirin or clopidogrel.
- Medical measures to reduce ICP (see Chapter 30).

Remember that in initial stages most patients with ICH will present with raised BP irrespective of presence of premorbid hypertension.

Surgical
- Controversial; early surgery reserved for younger patients with superficial lobar haematomas (within 1 cm of cortical surface) and a clot associated with significant mass effect leading to potential herniation; ICH in posterior (cerebellar) fossa associated with poor GCS ($\leq$13) or hydrocephalus.
- Hydrocephalus due to intraventricular extension of ICH or posterior fossa haematoma may require insertion of external ventricular drain (EVD).
- Surgery may also be needed for underlying AVM or aneurysm to reduce risk of rerupture.
- Not recommended in older patients $\geq$75 years of age; alert patient with minimal focal neurological deficit; large volume clot in dominant hemisphere; in those with poor GCS ($\leq$5) and in patients with deep haemorrhage, i.e. in basal ganglia, brainstem or thalamic haemorrhage.

COMPLICATIONS   Further clinical deterioration due to rebleeding, particularly in the early stages (within 24 h); hydrocephalus and increasing oedema around the clot.

PROGNOSIS   Death predominantly due to cerebral herniation; mortality rates around 40–45% over 30 days; better outcome with lobar haemorrhages.

DIFFERENTIAL DIAGNOSES   See Tables 14.3 and 33.1.

16   Stroke III: Subarachnoid haemorrhage

DEFINITION   Bleeding into the subarachnoid space, which lies between the arachnoid membrane and the pial surface of the brain and which usually is filled with CSF. May be spontaneous or secondary to trauma (the commonest cause).

EPIDEMIOLOGY
- Estimated annual incidence of aneurysmal subarachnoid haemorrhage (SAH) is 8–10/100 000.
- Aneurysmal SAH is rare in children; peak age is 55–60 years but up to 20% of cases occur in young adults.

AETIOLOGY
- Spontaneous SAH is a form of stroke.
- The commonest cause of spontaneous SAH is a ruptured intracranial aneurysm, accounting for 80% of cases.
- Other causes include rupture of arteriovenous malformations (6%); haemorrhage from tumours, including pituitary apoplexy; carotid or vertebral artery dissection; cerebral vasculitis; anticoagulant therapy and sickle cell disease.
- Approximately 10% of cases have no identifiable cause.

ASSOCIATIONS/RISK FACTORS
- Hypertension, smoking, drug abuse (cocaine and amphetamines), oral contraceptive use, pregnancy and parturition.
- *Genetic conditions*: Autosomal dominant polycystic kidney disease, Marfan's syndrome, fibromuscular dysplasia, familial intracranial aneurysm syndrome, Osler–Weber–Rendu syndrome and coarctation of the aorta.
- Bacterial endocarditis ('mycotic' aneurysms).

PATHOLOGY/PATHOGENESIS
- Aneurysmal SAH usually occurs due to rupture of saccular ('berry') aneurysms.
- Prevalence of Berry aneurysms is approximately 5%.
- Pathogenesis is not clearly established, strong association with smoking, hypertension and cerebrovascular arteriosclerotic disease.
- Risk may be further exacerbated by congenital predisposition due to defective muscular layer of arterial wall.
- Branching points of the major vessels of the circle of Willis are the commonest locations for aneurysm formation. A third of patients with SAH have multiple aneurysms.
- In addition to rupture, aneurysms may present with symptoms due to compression of adjacent neural structures.
- In infective endocarditis, 'mycotic' aneurysms develop due to damage of arterial wall due to infective emboli, the aneurysms are fusiform and friable. Mycotic aneurysms usually arise in the distal branches of vessels, most commonly those of the middle cerebral artery.

HISTORY
- Aneurysmal SAH commonly presents during exertion, coitus or parturition, but in over 30% of cases it occurs at rest or during sleep.

Headache:
- <u>Instantaneous onset</u>
- Severe 'the worst headache of my life' and of maximum severity from onset.
- Frequently described as a 'blow to the head'.
- Often associated with severe nausea and vomiting. Seizures may also occur.
- May persist for days.

Loss of consciousness:
- May occur at the time of rupture due to direct effect of haemorrhage or an associated intracerebral haematoma causing elevated ICP.
- May be transient or prolonged.
- In severe cases may lead to cardiorespiratory arrest and death.

Meningism:
- Photophobia and neck stiffness may be present.

Warning headache:
- Due to 'sentinel haemorrhage' that may precede major SAH in up to half of patients.
- Headache is of instantaneous onset but resolves relatively rapidly with no other major symptoms with the result that many patients do not seek medical attention.

Remember: SAH should be strongly suspected in any patient describing a severe headache of instantaneous onset even in the absence of other symptoms or signs of meningism.

Other symptoms:
- Irritation of lumbar nerve roots by SAH may cause lumbar back pain.
- Compression of third nerve by an enlarging aneurysm may cause diplopia and a ptosis.

EXAMINATION

Depressed level of consciousness/coma:
- Patients may be comatose from the outset or have a depressed level of consciousness.
- Document the Glasgow Coma Score (GCS).
- Grading by WFNS grade (Table 16.1).

Focal neurological deficits:
- Due to compression of adjacent neural structures by either the expanding aneurysm or an associated intracerebral haematoma.
- Basilar or posterior communicating artery aneurysm expansion may cause a *IIIrd nerve palsy*.
- Intracavernous sinus carotid aneurysms may present with opthalmoplegia (III, IV and VI nerves) and facial pain (V nerve, ophthalmic division).
- Internal carotid or anterior communicating artery aneurysms may compress the chiasm or optic nerves causing *visual field deficits* and the pituitary stalk causing *hypopituitarism*.

Table 16.1 WFNS grading of subarachnoid haemorrhage

Grade	GCS	Focal neurological deficit
I	15	Absent
II	13–14	Absent
III	13–14	Present
IV	7–12	Present or absent
V	<7	Present or absent

- Middle cerebral artery aneurysm may rupture into the parenchyma causing an intra-cerebral haematoma that compresses or damages the motor cortex or internal capsule causing a *hemiparesis*.

Meningism:
- Neck stiffness, 'nuchal rigidity' present on passive flexion of neck.
- Positive Kernig's sign (flex thigh with patient supine, then extend the knee, positive if causes pain in hamstrings preventing full extension). Usually seen >6 h following bleed.

Ocular haemorrhage:
- Seen on fundoscopy, often bilaterally.
- Preretinal (subhyaloid) haemorrhage, seen as blood obscuring retinal vessels in the region of optic disc, and/or vitreous haemorrhage (Terson's syndrome), seen as vitre-ous opacity.
- Occurs in approximately 10–20% of bleeds.
- In most cases, bleeding clears spontaneously but can lead to permanent visual loss.

Fever:
- Common.
- May be due to impairment of heat regulation due to hypothalamic damage or secondary infection.

Cardiovascular signs:
- Hypertension may be present.
- Cardiac arrhythmias may occur.
- In obtunded patients with raised ICP, Cushing's response (hypertension and bradycardia) may be seen.
- If a cardiac murmur is present on auscultation, consider infective endocarditis as a possible cause of SAH (mycotic aneurysm).

INVESTIGATIONS

Investigations are performed firstly to establish the diagnosis of SAH and then to identify the cause of the SAH.

To establish diagnosis:

CT head:
- Initial investigation if SAH is suspected following clinical evaluation.
- Will detect 95% of cases if done within 48 h of onset of symptoms.
- Location of the blood can localise the likely location of the aneurysm (Figure 16.1).
- Look also for complications of SAH, including intracerebral haematoma, intraventricular haemorrhage, cerebral infarction and hydrocephalus.
- Rarer causes of SAH such as tumours or AVMs may be seen.

Remember: CT head is the initial investigation of choice in patients with suspected SAH.

Lumbar puncture:
- If CT does not confirm SAH and the patient is alert without focal neurological signs, then a lumbar puncture should be performed >12 h after headache onset.
- CSF shows uniform blood staining in the first and third bottles with a xanthochromic (straw coloured) supernatant.
- Confirmation of blood breakdown products is usually confirmed on CSF spectro-photometry which identifies the presence of CSF bilirubin if SAH has occurred.
- If the patient is unconscious or with focal signs, an immediate neurosurgical referral is indicated without lumbar puncture.

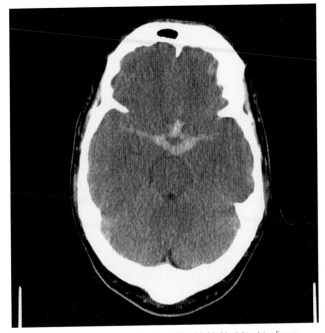

Figure 16.1 Axial CT Head showing acute subarachnoid blood (white) in right sylvian fissure, interhemispheric fissure and basal cisterns following rupture of an anterior communicating artery aneurysm.

MRI head:
- For patients with delayed presentation, MRI has a high sensitivity for detecting subarachnoid blood.
- Not helpful acutely (particularly <48 h due to lack of met-Hb).
- MR angiography may also enable detection of aneurysms (85% sensitivity), but is less reliable for detection of small aneurysms (<3 mm diameter).
- MR angiography is often used as screening test for unruptured aneurysms in patients at increased risk of aneurysm formation.

To identify cause (usually in neurosurgical unit):

Digital subtraction four-vessel angiography:
- 'Gold standard' investigation to identify aneurysm location.
- Other vascular lesions causing SAH such as AVMs are also identified using this technique.
- If initial angiography is negative, it is usually repeated at a later date as aneurysms may sometimes be obscured due to vasospasm of the artery from which it arises.

CT cerebral angiogram:
- Up to 95% sensitivity for aneurysm identification.
- Sometimes used to triage patients who may be suitable for endovascular coiling of the aneurysm.

MANAGEMENT

Management centres on control of the bleeding source, prevention and treatment of cerebral vasospasm and the treatment of other complications of SAH.

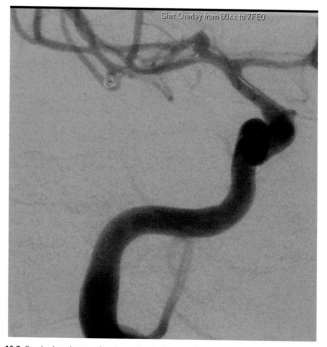

Figure 16.2 Cerebral angiogram showing coil embolisation of a small middle cerebral artery aneurysm.

Initial measures:
- Emergency medical management may include intubation and ventilation for comatose patients.
- ITU support and monitoring for severe SAH with NG feeding and urinary catheterisation to monitor fluid balance.
- Thromboprophylaxis with TED stockings and pneumatic calf compression.
- If seizures, load with intravenous phenytoin.
- Patients may require initial emergency neurosurgical intervention for early life-threatening complications of SAH such as hydrocephalus (treated with external ventricular or lumbar drainage) or a large intracerebral haematoma causing raised intra-cranial pressure, treated by craniotomy and haematoma evacuation.

Treatment of the aneurysm:
- Cerebral aneurysms are treated, when feasible, with endovascular coil embolisation.
- Endovascularly deployed platinum coils are placed in the aneurysm sac causing the lumen of the aneurysm to thrombose, obliterating it from the circulation (Figure 16.2).
- Where coiling cannot guarantee complete occlusion, a craniotomy (opening of the skull vault) is performed, the aneurysm is identified and a specialised clip placed across the neck of the aneurysm ('surgical clipping'), excluding it from the circulation.
- Treatment may be delayed for 2 weeks if severe vasospasm is present or if patient's initial neurological condition is very poor.

Prevention and treatment of cerebral vasospasm:
- Characterised by spasm of arteries within one or more arterial territories.
- Can follow SAH and, if severe, can leak to a delayed ischaemic neurological deficit (DIND) which can progress to permanent stroke.

- Rarely seen within the first 3 days following SAH.
- Usually develops between 3–21 days following SAH with a peak at 6–8 days.
- Risk factors for vasospasm include severity of bleed (blood load and clinical condition), hypovolaemia, a history of smoking or hypertension and increasing age.
- May be identified angiographically or using methods to evaluate cerebral blood flow such as xenon CT or MR perfusion/diffusion-weighted imaging.
- Bedside monitoring of middle cerebral artery blood flow using transcranial Doppler can also identify early vasospasm.
- Patients should be kept well hydrated, aiming for at least 3 L of fluid input a day.
- Antihypertensive therapy should be avoided.
- Nimodipine, a calcium channel blocker, has been shown to confer some prophylactic benefit in terms of improved neurological outcome and is routinely prescribed for 21 days following SAH.
- Lumbar CSF drainage also reduces the risk of vasospasm developing.
- In patients who develop symptomatic vasospasm, hyperdynamic therapy (known as 'triple H therapy': hypertension, hypervolaemia and haemodilution) is initiated. These patients should be managed in an intensive care setting. Plasma volume expansion is achieved with intravenous normal saline supplemented with colloid if required and haematocrit is kept between 25–33%. If the aneurysm is secured, pressors such as metaraminol or dobutamine are commenced to induce hypertension raising MAP by 15–20% or more.
- Refractory vasospasm can be treated with endovascular balloon angioplasty in some cases.

COMPLICATIONS

Stroke:
- Secondary to vasospasm.
- 25% develop a delayed ischaemic neurological deficit.
- 7% of patients die, 7% left with severe focal deficit.
- Commonly affects multiple vascular territories.

Hydrocephalus:
- 30% risk of early hydrocephalus requiring surgical intervention.
- May present as a delayed deterioration in the level of consciousness.
- Usually 'communicating' hydrocephalus but clots in the ventricle can cause 'obstructive' type.
- 10% require a VP shunt.
- May develop months or years after haemorrhage where onset may be insidious with progressive gait disturbance or cognitive decline.

Rebleeding:
- 4% risk of rebleeding in first 24 h.
- Untreated risk of rebleeding is 50% in 6 months.
- Poorer grade SAH has higher risk of rebleeding.
- Rebleeding carries a very high mortality (double initial bleed risk).
- Aneurysms treated with coiling are at greater risk of needing retreatment due to recurrent aneurysm formation.

Epilepsy:
- Occurs in 7–10%.
- Increased risk with higher blood load and cortical infarction.
- Associated with increased disability and poorer quality of life.

Hyponatraemia:
- Maintain on normal saline infusion to reduce risk of developing low sodium.
- Hyponatraemia due to either cerebral salt wasting or less commonly SIADH.
- Extracellular fluid volume is low in cerebral salt wasting and normal or elevated in SIADH.

- For cerebral salt wasting, avoid fluid restriction and supplement salt intake instead.
- Avoid rapid correction due to risk of central pontine myelinolysis.

Cardiac complications:
- ECG changes commonly following SAH.
- Ischaemic ECG changes may be seen, including ST changes.
- Elevated troponin in 20%, associated with reversible left ventricular dysfunction on echocardiogram: the 'stunned myocardium'.
- Ventricular fibrillation or other arrhythmias can occur.
- 'Neurogenic' pulmonary oedema can occur following SAH as a result of catecholamine surge due to sudden rise in ICP or hypothalamic injury.

> *Remember the list of complications above and consider them when approaching a patient with SAH who may have deteriorated subsequent to hospital admission.*

PROGNOSIS
- Fifteen per cent of patients with aneurysmal SAH die before reaching hospital.
- Overall mortality is around 50%.
- Thirty per cent of survivors have moderate to severe disability.
- Long-term cognitive dysfunction is common: memory and concentration problems, personality changes and executive dysfunction.
- Prognosis is worse in poor grade patients (GCS <7 at presentation), the elderly, patients with a heavy blood load on CT and in patients with posterior circulation (vertebrobasilar territory) aneurysms.

DIFFERENTIAL DIAGNOSES (TABLE 16.2)

Table 16.2 Differential diagnoses for SAH

Thunderclap headache	Benign orgasmic cephalalgia
Severe global headache with maximal intensity in <1 min	'Explosive' severe headache occurring during coitus or at the time of orgasm
Often associated with vomiting	May have history of migraine
No blood on CT and negative LP	Cannot reliably clinically distinguish from SAH, so require CT Head and LP to exclude SAH
Recurrent episodes occur	

17   Epilepsy

DEFINITION   Epilepsy is a disorder characterised by recurrent (≥2) unprovoked seizures. A seizure is a paroxysmal event marked by abnormal discharge of cerebral neurons resulting in alteration or impairment of consciousness, sensation or motor function.

Remember: A single seizure does not lead to a diagnosis of epilepsy.

EPIDEMIOLOGY
- Up to 5% of population may experience a single seizure; incidence similar in males and females.
- Generalised seizure disorders usually commence in childhood or adolescence. Focal seizures can start at any age and can be related in younger patients to hippocampal sclerosis. In older patients it may be associated with cerebrovascular disease or a structural abnormality (tumour).

AETIOLOGY   Aetiologies for the first seizure in adults include (i) idiopathic, (ii) acute or subacute neurological insult or injury due to stroke, head injury and infection (meningitis, encephalitis, subdural empyema and cerebral abscess), (iv) structural CNS diseases, including tumours (primary or metastatic), arteriovenous malformations and congenital CNS abnormalities, (iv) systemic disorders, including electrolyte disturbance (hyponatraemia or hypernatraemia, hypoglycaemia, hypercalcaemia, uraemia and magnesium level disturbances), hepatic encephalopathy and porphyria, (vi) toxin, illicit drug or medication related, including alcohol withdrawal or excess and (vii) eclampsia. In paediatric population, the first seizure may be due to a febrile episode or the so-called febrile convulsion, be it idiopathic or 'symptomatic or provoked' due to electrolyte disturbance, meningitis and so on.

CLASSIFICATION AND CHARACTERISTICS   This relies primarily on the mode of onset. Two main categories are primary generalised versus partial (focal) seizures with or without subsequent secondary generalisation.
Primary generalised seizures (40% of all seizures): Bilateral hemispheric symmetrical and synchronous discharge associated with loss of consciousness from the onset.
- *Generalised tonic–clonic (GTC) seizure (grand mal):* Sudden onset with loss of consciousness and initial tonic (stiffening of limbs) and then a clonic (jerking) phase; may be associated with urinary and/or faecal incontinence and tongue biting. In the postictal phase, patients are drowsy and confused with a gradual return of normal function.
- Tonic and clonic components can occur in isolation leading to tonic or clonic seizures, respectively.
- *Absence (petit mal):* Presents in childhood with episodes of transient (≤10 s) impairment of consciousness or pauses (staring episode) with minimal or no motor involvement. Three Hertz spike and wave activity on EEG. No postictal phase. Usual remission in teens.
- *Myoclonic seizures:* Characterised by sudden body jerks.
- *Atonic seizures:* Sudden transient loss of tone (flaccidity) leading to falls and high incidence of injury.
Partial seizures (around 50–60% of seizures): Attributed to seizure activity in one hemisphere or part of one hemisphere at the onset. Often occurs due to an underlying structural abnormality. Clinical features help localize area of onset, for example isolated limb jerking—contralateral motor strip arm region; lip smacking/chewing movements, olfactory or gustatory hallucination—contralateral medial temporal lobe; visual hallucination—occipital lobe and paraesthesia—contralateral somatosensory cortex. Classified as simple or complex, depending on whether consciousness is or is not impaired.

- *Simple partial seizure*: No impairment of consciousness, for example Jacksonian motor seizure.
- *Complex partial seizure*: With associated impairment of consciousness, often due to temporal lobe pathology; for example, hippocampal sclerosis leading to mesial temporal lobe epilepsy. Can be characterised by an aura (e.g. a rising epigastric sensation or olfactory or gustatory hallucinations) and the automatisms (e.g. lip smacking or chewing).
- *Partial seizure with secondary generalisation*: A seizure which is initially localization related (focal in onset and producing simple or complex phenomena) and then spreading to involve both hemispheres and hence evolving into, for example, a tonic–clonic episode.

> *Remember: The distinction between partial and generalised seizures is important clinically, not only for therapeutic purposes but also for the exams!*

ASSOCIATIONS/RISK FACTORS   Refer to Section 'Aetiology'. Certain factors can lower seizure threshold including photic stimulation (flashing lights) in certain forms of primary generalised epilepsy, hyperventilation, head injury and related posttraumatic seizures, systemic metabolic disturbances (as above) and infection of the CNS. lack of sleep, alcohol

PATHOLOGY/PATHOGENESIS   Seizures may occur due to an imbalance between excitatory and inhibitory components within cortical neurone networks leading to abnormal excitation.

Possible inherited predisposition to seizures as in primary generalised seizures. Some seizure syndromes like West and Lennox–Gestaut syndrome occur in childhood in association with structural CNS disease, for example tuberous sclerosis.

HISTORY
This is extremely important! An account of the events should be sought from a witness if available. See Chapter 6 regarding key points needing clarification in the history, particularly to distinguish seizures from syncope. 'Onset' of the sequence of events and establishing any possible compromise of consciousness often allows a clinical classification of seizures as above. Impairment of consciousness is reflected by the patient's partial or complete lack of memory about the episode. For example, a complex partial seizure with secondary generalisation to a tonic–clonic event may evolve as follows. A prodromal phase (not part of seizure and lasting hours to days) with a possible change in behaviour may be noted followed by an aura (part of the seizure, for example epigastric sensation and unusual smell, which is typically brief and may be associated with an altered level of awareness). With secondary generalization, patients may go on to lose consciousness with falling to the floor and witness tonic followed by clonic movements. Grunting noises, frothing at the mouth and rolling back of eyes may occur. Facial skin may be red or blue in colour (rather than deathly pale). Jerking movements may be seen usually for several minutes with possible associated urinary incontinence and tongue biting. The 'offset' of the seizure is typically abrupt followed by a period of marked confusion; the patient subsequently recalls that near clear memory was being in the Emergency Department. Question about any precipitating factors, for example alcohol use, with further questions directed towards other aetiological factors, for example systemic/metabolic or structural causes. ↓sleep, hypervent, flashing lights, alc, drugs

EXAMINATION
- In primary generalised epilepsy (idiopathic), clinical examination is usually normal between seizures (inter-ictal period). In partial seizures with or without generalisation, clinical examination may demonstrate a persistent focal deficit between seizures.
- If the seizure is witnessed by a doctor or a nurse, a detailed description (pre-event warning signs, onset, postural change, movements, colour of skin, whether eyes open or

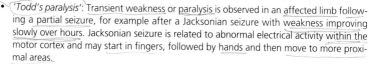

closed, duration of event, associated features (incontinence) and offset) should be noted in a seizure chart.

- In the immediate 'postictal' phase, patients may be drowsy and confused following a GTC seizure.
- 'Todd's paralysis': Transient weakness or paralysis is observed in an affected limb following a partial seizure, for example after a Jacksonian seizure with weakness improving slowly over hours. Jacksonian seizure is related to abnormal electrical activity within the motor cortex and may start in fingers, followed by hands and then move to more proximal areas.

INVESTIGATIONS In an adult presenting with a first seizure, direct tests towards establishing a possible underlying cause, particularly if no provoking factors are obvious, for example alcohol withdrawal (refer to aetiologies). Test should include the following:

- *Blood tests*: FBC, U & E, serum glucose level (also fingerstick glucose), calcium, magnesium, LFT and blood and urine toxin levels if suspected drug or alcohol abuse.
- *Imaging studies*: Perform a CT with or without contrast to look for a structural lesion. This may be followed up with an MRI with or without gadolinium to assess for structural lesions (neoplasm, arteriovenous malformations or cavernomas). Repeat imaging studies may be needed.
- *EEG*: May be performed to help in classifying seizure type.

> *Remember: In an adult presenting with a first seizure, imaging studies starting with a CT of brain with or without contrast is an important part of diagnostic work up to exclude a structural lesion like neoplasm, abscess or vascular malformations.*

MANAGEMENT

- *Treatment*: Commence after a patient has suffered two or more seizures within a 2-year period.
- Choice of first line antiepileptic drug (AED) varies according to the aetiology and classification of seizure type.

> *Remember: There are many different anticonvulsant drugs to choose from and the following are given by way of example only. In the United Kingdom, AEDs usually have approval as mono or adjunctive therapies or both and for partial, myoclonic or tonic–clonic seizures or a combination of these. The British National Formulary (BNF) provides further information.*

- *Primary generalised seizures*: Sodium valproate, Levetiracetam or Lamotrigine are commonly used as first line agent, but alternatives are available. Childhood absence epilepsy can be treated with sodium valproate.
- *Partial* seizures with or without secondary generalisation: Carbamazepine, lamotrigine or levetiracetam are commonly used as first line drugs, but alternatives are available.
- *Phenytoin*: An effective drug widely used in neurosurgical practice and in patients presenting acutely with status epilepticus (SE) (see Appendix 1). Also used as a short-term prophylactic drug (for a week) to prevent early ($\leq$7 days) posttraumatic seizures in high-risk patients (with acute subdural, extradural or intracerebral haematoma; depressed skull fracture with intraparenchymal injury or intraparenchymal contusions, particularly involving temporal lobe).

Remember: Phenytoin, although an effective AED, is not usually suitable for long-term maintenance therapy owing to its side effects profile.

- *Examples of newer effective and well tolerated AEDs*: Levetiracetam, topiramate, zonisamide and lacosamide and others.
- *The goal*: Achieve seizure freedom with one (monotherapy) well-tolerated drug. The basic treatment principle is to increase drug dose as tolerated until seizure control is achieved or maximum drug dose reached or unacceptable side effects occur.
- If seizures are still uncontrolled, start a second AED and gradually increase to target dose before withdrawing the first agent (e.g. over 6–8 weeks). Ideally only use dual therapy if all appropriate drugs have failed to control seizures singly at their maximum tolerated dose.
- Phenytoin, phenobarbitone and carbamazepine are liver enzyme inducers and therefore increase the elimination rate for contraceptive pills and other drugs metabolised by the liver, for example phenytoin.

Remember: To address the issue of 'the oestrogen-containing pill' and liver enzyme-inducing AEDs, advise an increase in contraceptive pill dosage with use of barrier contraception when starting treatment of women of childbearing age with AEDs. Teratogenicity is also a risk in this age group and women should be counselled; avoid polytherapy and reduce dose to the minimum effective dose to reduce this risk. High-dose folic acid (5 mg/day) is prescribed preconceptually and throughout pregnancy to reduce incidence of neural tube defects, a particular concern with sodium valproate.

- All AEDs can potentially lead to sedation. The following are some of the important side effects of common AEDs:
  o *Phenytoin*: Serum levels are measured to monitor drug dosage. Signs of toxicity are nystagmus, ataxia, diplopia, dysarthria, CNS depression and confusion. Other side effects at therapeutic levels are rash, cognitive decline, acne and hirsutism, gingival hypertrophy, osteomalacia (antagonises vitamin D), blood dyscrasias and hepatic dysfunction.
  o *Sodium valproate*: Weight gain, reversible hair loss, liver dysfunction, hyperammonaemia and tremor.
  o *Carbamazepine*: Rash, transient diplopia, ataxia, GI upset, SIADH (with hyponatraemia) and haematological effects rarely leading to agranulocytosis and aplastic anaemia.
  o *Lamotrigine*: Rash, diplopia and somnolence. Its metabolism can be affected by other AEDs, for example sodium valproate increases its half-life significantly.

PROGNOSIS
- Depends on the underlying aetiology and on the particular epilepsy syndrome; most generalised epilepsies will achieve remission in early adult life.
- *Mortality rates*: Higher by 1.6–9 times compared to general population.
- Death may be due to underlying disorder (e.g. brain tumour); sudden unexpected death in epilepsy (SUDEP); accidents during an epileptic attack, for example drowning; status epilepticus. SUDEP (accounting for up to 17% of deaths in this population), defined as sudden unexpected death occurring in an epileptic patient with the event not happening during a seizure and followed by a normal post-mortem examination probably has a multifactorial mechanism including bradyarrhythmias and respiratory depression.

DIFFERENTIAL DIAGNOSES   Refer to Chapter 6. Do not forget non-epileptic attacks disorder as a differential (seek expert neurology opinion).

MANAGEMENT OF STATUS EPILEPTICUS (SEE APPENDIX 1)

Other points of note:

- Advise patients to inform Driving and Vehicle Licensing Authority (DVLA) subsequent to a seizure. Activities like swimming should be avoided and patients should be told not to bathe alone. Medically refractory seizure disorder, for example due to mesial temporal sclerosis-related epilepsy, may be amenable to surgical treatment, for example amygdalohippocampectomy. Detailed evaluation takes place prior to surgery, including imaging studies (MRI, fMRI and PET scan), EEG, including video-EEG and recordings from invasive intracranial electrodes, and neuropsychological assessment.
- *Febrile seizures of childhood*: Very common and associated with fever (e.g. related to vaccination) and not accompanied by an acute neurological illness. The risk of developing epilepsy subsequent to a simple febrile seizure is 1%; anticonvulsants not routinely prescribed in these cases.
- *West syndrome (a seizure disorder appearing in the first year of life)*: Characterised by recurrent flexion of trunk and limbs (also known as infantile spasms). Associated with mental retardation and can be secondary to tuberous sclerosis. Interictal hypsarrhythmia on EEG. Responds to ACTH or corticosteroids.
- *Lennox–Gastaut syndrome (a disorder arising in childhood)*: Characterised by recurrent atonic seizures or drop attacks, mental retardation and can be often medically refractory. Treat with sodium valproate. Corpus callosotomy is another option for reducing atonic seizures.

18   Multiple sclerosis

DEFINITION   Multiple sclerosis (MS) is an inflammatory disease of the CNS characterised by *multiple* episodes of demyelination separated in *time and space*.

> Remember: A single episode of demyelination should not lead to a diagnosis of MS as implied by the above definition.

EPIDEMIOLOGY   Affects approximately 1 in 1000 people in the United Kingdom. F:M = 1.5–2:1. Onset is typically between 20 and 40 years of age. Common in people of northern European ancestry.

AETIOLOGY   The exact cause unknown and may occur due to a complex interaction between environmental and genetic factors.
- *Genetic factors*: Relative risk for a first-degree relative is two–four times higher than background risk. HLA-DRB1 is a chromosomal locus consistently associated with susceptibility to MS.
- *Other aetiological factors*: Viruses, molecular mimicry and auto-immunological mechanisms.

ASSOCIATIONS/RISK FACTORS   Migration to high-risk areas in northern latitudes before 15 years of age increases the risk of developing MS. MS relapses can be associated with inter-current infection, while a reduction in relapse rate is noted during pregnancy.

PATHOLOGY/PATHOGENESIS
- Perivascular infiltration of lymphocytes (T cells) and macrophages in brain parenchyma, brainstem, optic nerve and spinal cord; thought to be mediated by activated T cells.
- *Plaque* (*characterised by demyelination with preservation of axons*): This pathological hallmark occurs more commonly in periventricular white matter and the corpus callosum.
- CNS demyelination causes slowing or interruption of conduction through the brain and spinal cord as seen on neurophysiological testing.

> Remember: Demyelinated plaques are the pathological hallmark of MS and occur commonly in periventricular white matter and corpus callosum.

HISTORY   Patients may report symptoms of visual, sensory, motor, coordination, bladder or sexual dysfunction with or without disturbance in cognition or mood. Principal subtypes are relapsing/remitting MS (RRMS), where symptoms of relapse are separated over time and anatomical location (optic neuritis, disequilibrium etc.) with recovery or partial recovery in between; secondary progressive MS (SPMS), where a period of relapse is followed by relentless progression producing ever-increasing disability; and primary progressive MS (PPMS), where patients relentlessly deteriorate from outset without a proceeding history of relapses or recovery. About 50–75% of RRMS patients will enter the SPMS phase 10–20 years post the onset of first symptom. PPMS is much rarer than the other subtypes; commoner in males with a greater effect on limb and bladder dysfunction.
- *Visual*: Optic neuritis (a common initial complaint with pain on eye movement and mild to severe visual loss including colour vision typically involving only one eye at a time; full or partial recovery usually occurs over months), Uhthoff's phenomenon (a temporary worsening of neurological symptoms such as visual loss in multiple sclerosis provoked by an increase in body temperature, for example during a fever or a hot bath).

- *Sensory*: Paraesthesia and numbness affecting the limbs or trunk; Lhermitte's phenomenon, an electric shock-like sensation down the back and limbs produced by neck flexion due to a demyelinating plaque in the cervical cord; trigeminal neuralgia (TN).
- *Motor*: Limb weakness and stiffness.
- *Brainstem/cerebellum*: Diplopia related to IIIrd, IVth or VIth nerve involvement or due to an internuclear ophthalmoplegia (INO); vertigo; dizziness; ataxia and tremor.
- *Sphincter and sexual function*: These symptoms typically parallel limb symptoms due to cord involvement. Urinary urgency and frequency with retention (UMN-type unstable bladder); erectile dysfunction and impotence.
- *Others*: Fatigue (a prominent symptom), cognitive deficits, pseudo-bulbar affect; euphoria and depression.

The Kurtzke Expanded Disability Status Scale is a rating scale of clinical disease severity. A score of (0–10) is assigned to the patient's clinical status with mobility as the major determinant.

EXAMINATION

- *Eyes*: Relative afferent pupillary defect (RAPD), central scotoma and colour disturbance (red desaturation) may be seen with optic neuritis; optic atrophy (pale discs) commonly seen post recurrent or unresolved optic neuritis; ataxic nystagmus is seen with unilateral or bilateral INO.
- *Motor*: UMN signs (spasticity, hyperreflexia and up-going plantars).
- *Sensory*: Impairment of light touch, pinprick, joint position or vibration sense. A truncal sensory level may be seen due to MS-related inflammation of the spinal cord—transverse myelitis.
- *Cerebellum*: Nystagmus, dysarthria, intention tremor, dysdiadochokinesia, limb, truncal and gait ataxia.

INVESTIGATIONS

- *MRI with and without Gadolinium*: Multiple T2 hyperintensities (enhancing and non-enhancing) especially in periventricular region and corpus callosum reflect white matter change (Figure 18.1). Active inflammatory lesions enhance with Gadolinium.

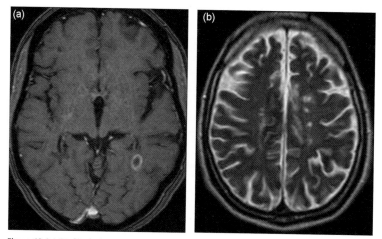

Figure 18.1 MRI of brain demonstrating demyelinating plaques as represented by (a) enhancing white matter lesion on axial T1-weighted image with Gadolinium (b) hyperintense lesions on axial T2-weighted image.

- *CSF*: Mild lymphocytic pleocytosis, normal glucose and normal to mildly elevated protein, oligoclonal bands on protein electrophoresis in CSF but not in serum due to intrathecal immunoglobulin synthesis (in 95% of MS cases, however non-specific).
- *Neurophysiology*: Delayed VEP (50–80% sensitivity) and SSEP are particularly useful at detecting clinically silent lesions.

> *Remember: There is no clear correlation between the appearance on MRI and patient's clinical status. Also make note of the point regarding presence of oligoclonal bands on protein electrophoresis in CSF but not in serum.*

MANAGEMENT

> *Remember: Steroid (high-dose pulsed methylprednisolone IV or oral) during acute exacerbations hastens recovery with no effect on the degree of recovery, frequency of relapse or overall disease progression.*

- *Immunomodulators*: Decrease in frequency and severity of relapses in RRMS may be achieved by using immunomodulatory drugs [(i.e. interferon beta-1a, interferon beta-1b and glatiramer acetate (Copaxone)].
- Natalizumab or Alemtuzumab (monoclonal antibodies) dramatically reduce relapse rates in aggressive RRMS but carry significant risk.
- Mitoxantrone, an immunosuppressor, may be used for reducing neurological disability and/or the frequency of clinical relapses in patients with SPMS and worsening RRMS, although toxicity limits its use.
- Other treatments employed are symptom improving rather than disease modifying—spasticity (Baclofen), fatigue (Amantadine), unstable bladder (oxybutynin and intermittent self-catheterisation), TN or Lhermitte's (Carbamazepine), mood disorder (antidepressants) and, importantly, multidisciplinary support including PT/OT and MS nurse.

COMPLICATIONS   Side effects from drugs, for example flu-like symptoms and local irritation from interferons; aspiration pneumonia, pressure sores and so on in immobile MS patients; slight increase in seizure risk.

PROGNOSIS   Up to 10% have milder form with no significant disease progression; life expectancy reduced by between 5–7 years; men with PPMS have the poorest prognosis.

DIFFERENTIAL DIAGNOSES (TABLE 18.1)   A wide differential based on presentation:
Other differentials: Inflammatory disease (SLE, sarcoidosis and Behcet's disease) and infectious (syphilis, HIV and lyme). Carry out appropriate blood tests, including autoimmune screen and relevant serology for infectious diseases.

Table 18.1 Differential diagnoses for MS with distinguishing features

Clinical conditions	How to exclude it (distinguishing features)
Acute disseminated encephalomyelitis (ADEM)	Monophasic illness with multiple areas of demyelination separated in space but not time, unlike MS. Enquire about a recent history of viral illness which is more common in ADEM
Structural lesion, for example tumours causing spinal cord compression or optic neuritis	Appropriate imaging (MRI) of spinal cord or brain

Devic's disease or neuromyelitis optica	Thought to be a variant of MS with myelitis and optic neuritis. MRI and blood test for Aquaporin 4 antibody
Brainstem syndrome related to vascular or infective aetiology (encephalitis)	History, imaging (MRI) and CSF examination
Amyotrophic lateral sclerosis	Presence of LMN as well as UMN signs with typically normal MRI of the brain

19   Parkinson's disease and other related syndromes

DEFINITION   Parkinson's disease (PD) is a common slowly progressive bradykinetic neuro-degenerative disorder predominantly affecting people over the age of 60. The principal motor symptoms are due to degeneration of the dopaminergic nigrostriatal pathway. PD acquires its name from James Parkinson, an apothecary surgeon, who produced a monograph in 1817 entitled *An Essay on the Shaking Palsy* in which he described six people with a hitherto unrecognised neurological disorder. The diagnosis is clinical and based upon having two or more of the following features: tremor, rigidity, bradykinesia and postural instability (see below).

EPIDEMIOLOGY
- The incidence of PD rises steeply with age with median age of onset being 60 years.
- Affects 1% of the population over the age of 60 with 10% of patients, however, developing symptoms before the age of 50. Slightly more common in men than in women (1.2:1).

AETIOLGY
Sporadic:
- Only a few environmental causes have so far been identified.
- Never smokers are twice as likely to develop PD. Low caffeine intake slightly increases the risk of developing PD.
- Certain environmental toxins, such as exposure to the designer drug MPTP, and carbon monoxide poisoning can produce a parkinsonian disorder but this is not the same as idiopathic Parkinson's disease.

> *Remember: The increased risk of developing PD in non-smokers and low caffeine drinkers is not understood. Although the explanation could be that nicotine is neuro-protective, an alternative explanation is that PD occurs more commonly in people with low pre-morbid novelty seeking personality traits.*

Genetic:
- Mendelian-type genetic mutations account for approximately 5% of patients with Parkinson's disease in the United Kingdom. The most common autosomal dominant mutations producing PD are in the gene LRRK-2.
- The most common autosomal recessive mutations causing parkinsonism are in the parkin gene.

PATHOLOGY
- Motor symptoms in PD are due to the degeneration of the dopaminergic projection extending from the cell bodies in the substantia nigra of the mid-brain to the terminal innervation of the striatum (putamen and caudate nucleus) in the basal forebrain.
- The Lewy Body, composed of misfolded synuclein, found in the perikarya of the dopamine neurones of the substantia nigra is the histopathological hallmark.
- Extensive pathology in other monoaminergic systems, outside the dopaminergic nigrostriatal pathway, and the change in cholinergic and glutamatergic pathways are also seen.

> *Remember: Lewy Body is the histopathological hallmark of PD.*

HISTORY
- The onset is typically in one or the other upper limbs, typically asymmetric (due to greater degeneration of the contralateral nigrostriatal pathway).

- Tremor, difficulty with fine finger movement, micrographia, difficulty turning in bed and reduced walking speed.
- Approximately 5% of patients present with what appears to be a frozen shoulder.
- Often at presentation, patients complain of slowing with activities of daily living, such as washing or dressing.

EXAMINATION

- Tremor is typically asymmetric, present at rest and improved by action, increased by mental strain and is of a 4–6 Hz frequency.
- Rigidity refers to an increase in limb tone i.e. equal throughout the range of movement (in contrast to spasticity, which demonstrates a catch on tone testing). Typically asymmetric.
- Bradykinesia refers to not only a reduction in amplitude and speed of movement but also to fatiguing over time, as seen on repeated finger tapping.
- Stooped posture.
- In the early stage of disease, a reduction in unilateral arm swing is seen on walking. Subsequently, gait is stooped and shuffling and may demonstrate festination and freezing.
- Postural instability may be revealed by unsteadiness or occasional stumbling on corner turning with the patient taking several steps backwards or needing to be caught on draw testing.

Remember: TRAP (tremor, rigidity, akinesia or bradykinesia and postural instability) in PD.

INVESTIGATIONS

- No single diagnostic test for PD.
- *Blood*: To rule out hypothyroidism or hyperthyroidism.
- *MRI or CT brain scan*: To rule out structural causes of parkinsonism, such as normal pressure hydrocephalus (see Chapter 29) or extensive white matter changes as may be seen in vascular parkinsonism.
- Functional neuroimaging (Figure 19.1) including ^{18}F-dopa PET scanning or DAT imaging to demonstrate loss of dopamine terminal innervation in the putamen may be available in some centres and supports a diagnosis but will not distinguish between PD and atypical parkinsonian disorders, which share destruction of the nigrostriatal pathway as part of their pathology.

Remember: Diagnosis is clinical and depends upon a careful history and examination, particularly to exclude other causes of parkinsonism (Table 19.1).

MANAGEMENT
Medical:

- Dopaminergic therapy using either a dopamine (D2) agonist drug or the *L-Dopa* to improve stiffness, slowness and tremor.
- Dopamine agonists come in both ergot and non-ergot forms. The ergot-derived agonists have fallen out of favour because of risks of lung, retroperitoneal and cardiac fibrosis. The non-ergot agonists include *Ropinirole, Pramipexole and Rotigotine* (given via a transdermal patch).
- *L-Dopa* is a prodrug which can cross the blood–brain barrier and is converted to dopamine in the pre-synaptic terminal. It is combined with a peripheral decarboxylase inhibitor to prevent peripheral breakdown and therefore reduce the quantity required.

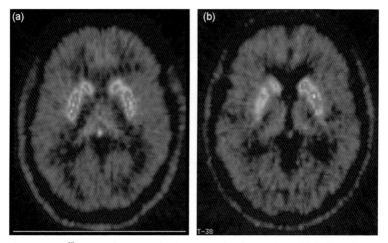

Figure 19.1 An ^{18}F-PET scan from a control and a patient with Parkinson's disease. (a) The figure shows an ^{18}F-PET scan from a healthy control, normal ^{18}F-dopa uptake is shown in caudate and putamen and the scan demonstrates normal striatal dopamine terminal plexus integrity. (b) This shows asymmetrically reduced ^{18}F-dopa uptake in caudate and putamen in a patient with PD.

Table 19.1 Differential diagnoses of Parkinson's disease with differentiating features

Condition	Features that differentiate from idiopathic PD
Progressive supranuclear palsy (PSP)	More rapid progression, falls within 2 years of onset of symptoms, lack of L-Dopa response, extraocular eye signs (supranuclear gaze palsy), dysarthria and early dementia. MRI may show atrophy of the mid-brain
Multiple system atrophy (MSA)	More rapid progression, falls within 2 years of onset of symptoms and lack of L-Dopa response, may demonstrate autonomic features (MSA-P) or may demonstrate cerebellar features (MSA-C). MRI may show cerebellar atrophy
Corticobasal degeneration (CBD)	More rapid progression, falls within 2 years of onset of symptoms and lack of L-Dopa response. May also demonstrate alien limb phenomena, myoclonic jerks and early dementia. MRI may show asymmetric cortical atrophy
Lewy Body dementia (LBD) (Chapter 29)	More rapid progression, falls within 2 years of onset of symptoms and lack of L-Dopa response. Dementia occurs within 2 years, apparent daily fluctuations in cognitive functioning and visual hallucinations
Vascular parkinsonism	May show lack of progression or stepwise progression, typically demonstrates a lack of L-Dopa response. Tends to be more symmetric and often presents with lower body (particularly gait) disturbance. MRI shows extensive small vessel white matter disease

- Other commonly employed medical therapies include monoamine oxidase inhibitors (*MAOI type B: Rasagiline or Selegiline*), glutamate antagonists (Amantadine), anticholinergics (Trihexyphenidyl) and sometimes beta-blockers for tremor.
- If severe motor complications arise, additional medical therapy options include subcutaneous Apomorphine (a potent dopamine agonist) or Jejunal-infused duodopa.

Surgical:

- *Deep brain stimulation (DBS) surgery* with targeting of the region of the subthalamic nucleus: employed in less than 3% of patients to improve a drug-resistant parkinsonian action tremor and/or motor complications, including L-Dopa-induced dyskinesias and 'on/off' fluctuations.

Supportive:

- Regular follow-up care by a specialist in Parkinson's disease (typically a neurologist or elderly care physician) plus a multi-disciplinary team approach, including PD nurses, physiotherapists, occupational therapists and psychiatrists.

COMPLICATIONS   Although a slowly progressive disease that for many years is typically highly responsive to dopaminergic therapy, after 5–10 years the majority of patients develop the so-called motor complications (L-Dopa-induced dyskinesias, end of dose deterioration, 'on/off' fluctuations, freezing of gait and falls). These motor complications can be very difficult to manage. In addition, non-motor symptoms occur with increasing frequency, including loss of smell, mood disorders, executive dysfunction and dementia, autonomic disturbance (postural hypotension, urinary frequency and hesitancy, constipation and swallowing difficulties), hypophonia and sleep disturbance.

PROGNOSIS   The commonest cause for nursing home placement is dementia and postural instability with falls. Mean survival from symptom onset is 15 years.

> *Remember: PD is a relentlessly progressive disorder with no therapy licensed to slow the progression of the disease. Medical treatments, therefore, are symptom improving only.*

DIFFERNTIAL DIAGNOSES

> *Remember: PSP, MSA, CBD and LBD collectively may be termed as the atypical parkinsonian disorders. All these disorders show changes on ^{18}Dopa PET and DAT imaging and, therefore, the distinction from PD and also from each other is largely based upon clinical features.*

20   Other movement disorders

DEFINITION   Movement disorders are typically divided into two forms: hyperkinetic and hypokinetic.

Hypokinetic movement disorders include the akinetic rigid syndromes discussed in Chapter 19. *Hyperkinetic* disorders are also called dyskinesias. There are five forms of dyskinesias, including tremor, dystonia, chorea, tics and myoclonus. The body region distribution of hyperkinetic movement disorders vary, for example can be focal, multi-focal, generalised or unilateral. The above describes phenomenology, i.e. the type of involuntary movement and its distribution as described or seen. A further important step is to consider aetiology.

AETIOLOGY   Hyperkinetic movement disorders are considered to be either of the following:
- *Primary*: Isolated movement disorders, i.e. without cognitive decline, epilepsy or other neurological features; not progressive and inherited, so check family history.
- *Secondary*: An identifiable secondary cause such as brain injury, infection, toxic or drug exposure; may improve with removal of provoking cause.
- *Heredodegenerative*: As part of a generalised degenerative process; additional psychiatric and systemic problems.
- *Psychogenic*: History of psychological disturbance and medically unexplained symptoms.

> *Remember: It is important to rule out treatable causes of hyperkinetic movement disorders like Wilson's disease and dopa-responsive dystonia, which although rare are amenable to treatment. The age at the onset of symptom, precipitating and relieving factors, drug exposure, family history and other associated features with examination findings detailing the distribution and type of hyperkinetic movement seen will narrow the differential diagnoses.*

Tremor

Tremor is easily recognised as a rhythmic sinusoidal movement. When describing tremor it is useful to detail whether present with rest (in Parkinson's disease), posture (e.g. holding the arms outstretched in front of the patient, as in the so-called essential tremor) and with action (e.g. drinking from a cup). Important causes of postural tremor include physiological tremor, anxiety, hyperthyroidism, certain medications, alcohol and caffeine use, essential (familial) tremor and Wilson's disease.

Isolated kinetic (action) tremors can be seen with structural abnormalities of the brainstem and cerebellar connections, as in multiple sclerosis, vascular disease or secondary tumours.

Essential (familial) tremor

DEFINITION   Essential tremor (ET) is a syndromic diagnosis. It typically presents as a symmetrical postural tremor and often has an autosomal dominant fashion of inheritance.

EPIDEMIOLOGY   Bimodal onset (childhood and late life onset), men and women are equally affected. Prevalence is approximately 300 per 100 000.

AETIOLOGY   A family history is found in approximately 50% of cases (autosomal dominant inheritance).

HISTORY   Typically a fine distal symmetrical upper limb tremor, starting gradually and worsening over time. Voice tremor may be present. Often marked improvement with alcohol is seen.

INVESTIGATIONS   There are no diagnostic tests. Important to exclude hyperthyroidism or drugs causing tremor.

MANAGEMENT   *Medical*: First line therapy—propranolol or primidone or a combination of both; second line therapy—gabapentin or topiramate. *Surgical*: Severe functionally impairing ET resistant to medical therapies may be suitable for and respond to deep brain stimulation surgery.

Chorea

DEFINITION   Described as brief irregular purposeless movements flowing from one body part to another. People appear restless or fidgety. Chorea is often generalised but may be confined to one side of the body (hemichorea) typically due to a structural cause within the contralateral basal ganglia.

AETIOLOGY
- *Genetic*: Huntington's disease (autosomal dominant), Wilson's disease (autosomal recessive) and other inherited causes.
- *Autoimmune*: Systemic lupus erythematosus, antiphospholipid syndrome and Sydenham's chorea.
- Infections, medications (L-Dopa-induced dyskinesias) and metabolic (thyroid dysfunction and chorea gravidarum).

Huntington's disease (HD)

DEFINITION   An autosomal dominant degenerative disease characterised by progressive behavioural disturbance, dementia and chorea.

EPIDEMIOLOGY   HD affects 4–8/100 000; males and females are affected equally.

HISTORY   Motor onset is variable but usually in the fourth decade; psychiatric symptoms, particularly disinhibited behaviour, may be the first feature. Abnormalities of eye movement, gait, upper motor neurone signs and tics may be seen along with chorea.

INVESTIGATIONS   Genetic testing (HD is a triplet repeat disorder with mutation in the Huntingtin gene on chromosome 4). MRI may show caudate nucleus atrophy.

MANAGEMENT   Medical (tetrabenazine may be used to improve chorea) and multi-disciplinary team approach (psychiatry, genetic counselling for family members, physiotherapy and occupational therapy).

Wilson's disease

DEFINITION   Wilson's disease is a condition characterised by a defect in copper metabolism leading to accumulation of copper in liver and basal ganglia.

Remember: Although rare, it is treatable. With treatment, symptoms may be reversed or progression halted. If left untreated, it is fatal.

EPIDEMIOLOGY   Rare with a prevalence of 30 per million, onset is usually in teens but can be up to 50 years.

AETIOLOGY   An autosomal recessive condition due to a mutation in the copper-transporting gene on chromosome 13.

HISTORY AND EXAMINATION   Childhood presentation (mean age 11 years) is typically with acute liver failure or signs of chronic liver disease. Presentation in the late teens is typically neurological and consists of tremor, dystonia, parkinsonism, cerebellar signs and gait disturbance accompanied by psychiatric manifestations.

INVESTIGATIONS
- *Serum copper and caeruloplasmin blood tests*: Caeruloplasmin, a copper-transporting protein, is low with low serum copper levels; raised 24 h urinary copper excretion (greater sensitivity than blood testing).
- Slit-lamp examination of the eyes demonstrates Kayser–Fleischer rings in 100% of patients with neurological manifestations.
- An MRI of the brain may show symmetrical high signal changes in the basal ganglia.

MANAGEMENT   Copper chelating drugs (penicillamine and trientine) with close monitoring to demonstrate copper removal.

Dystonia

DEFINITION   Defined as involuntary co-contraction of agonist and antagonist muscles, leading to sustained abnormal postures of the affected body part. Typically, the abnormal postures are not fixed and slow writhing movements can occur. Dystonic tremor may accompany dystonic posturing and is distinguished from essential tremor by its more jerky and variable amplitude appearance.

Dystonia can be classified by the distribution of body parts affected:
- Focal dystonia (e.g. cervical dystonia and torticollis).
- Segmental dystonia (two or more contiguous body parts).
- Hemidystonia (dystonia affecting one side of the body).
- Generalised dystonia (two or more contiguous body parts affected plus the trunk).

AETIOLOGY
- *Primary dystonia*: Dystonia is seen with or without tremor and the cause is typically genetic or a secondary cause such as brain injury or toxic exposure is found.
- *Heredodegenerative dystonia*: Occurring in the context of a neurodegenerative condition.
- *Paroxysmal dystonia*: Episodic attacks of dystonia without clinical signs in between.
- Psychogenic dystonia.

INVESTIGATIONS   In *primary dystonia* there is an underlying genetic mutation such as DYT1. *Secondary dystonia* may demonstrate structural changes on MRI. Wilson's disease (as above), a heredodegenerative dystonia, shows abnormalities on copper studies.

MANAGEMENT
- *Medical*: Drug treatments, for example Trihexyphenidyl, and Botulinum toxin injections are treatment of choice in cervical dystonia.
- In severe generalised dystonia refractory to medical or Botulinum toxin therapy, deep brain stimulation surgery may bring marked improvement.

> *Remember: Patients below the age of 30 presenting with dystonia not due to an identifiable secondary cause should receive a course of L-Dopa in case of the so-called dopa-responsive dystonia, which is highly responsive to treatment.*

21   Central nervous system infections: Meningitis

DEFINITION   Infection and/or inflammation of the pia and arachnoid and the cerebrospinal fluid that they enclose. It therefore involves both the cranial and spinal compartments.

EPIDEMIOLOGY

Neonate: Group B streptococcus, followed by *Escherichia coli* and *Listeria monocytogenes*. Increased risk with prematurity, prolonged membrane rupture, traumatic delivery, congenital malformations and acquired respiratory, gastroenterological or umbilical infections.

1–3 months: *Streptococcus pneumoniae*.

3 months–3 years: Haemophilus influenzae type B, related to nasopharyngeal colonisation.

Children and young adults: *Neisseria meningitidis*. Nasopharyngeal colonisation leads to haematogenous dissemination and meningitis, occurring in epidemics. Low complement increases risk.

Elderly and alcoholics: *S. pneumoniae*. Increased risk with age-dependent reduction in immunity.

Posttraumatic: *S. pneumoniae*, representing the normal flora of the mastoid, ear, nose and cranial sinuses. Increased risk with cerebrospinal fluid fistula.

Postneurosurgical: *Staphylococcus epidermidis* and *Staphylococcus aureus*, Enterobacteriaecae, *Pseudomonas* species and pneumococci.

Immunocompromised patients: *S. pneumoniae*, *Cryptococcus neoformans* and *Mycobacterium* tuberculosis.

AETIOLOGY   Bacterial (*Haemophilus influenzae*, *S. pneumoniae*, *N. meningitidis*, *L. monocytogenes*, in descending order, are the commonest bacterial organisms), viral and fungal.

PATHOLOGY/PATHOGENESIS   Bacteria in cerebrospinal fluid excite an inflammatory reaction in the vascular pia, leading to exudation of blood proteins and migration of neutrophils. Thrombosis of superficial veins causes brain infarction. Accumulation of exudate obstructs flow of cerebrospinal fluid, causing hydrocephalus. Penetration of the arachnoid causes subdural inflammation and effusions. Structures in the subarachnoid space, such as cranial nerves, are inflamed and damaged; deafness (damage to VIIIth nerve in the basal cisterns) is a common complication of meningitis in children. Retrograde spread of infection and inflammation in the cerebrospinal fluid causes ventriculitis.

HISTORY   Fever, severe headache, drowsiness, vomiting, confusion, coma, generalised seizures (particularly in neonates, infants and young children), features related to concurrent infections, immunosuppression and trauma.

EXAMINATION
- *Signs of meningeal irritation:* Neck stiffness on forward flexion, inability to completely extend the legs (Kernig's sign).
- Bulging fontanelles in neonates and infants.
- *Petechial and purpuric rash with circulatory collapse:* Characteristic of the Waterhouse–Friderichsen syndrome in meningococcal meningitis. Concomitant evidence of disseminated intravascular coagulation and shock supports this diagnosis.
- Look for sepsis elsewhere, for example ears, throat and upper respiratory tract, lung and heart valves, and for clues to cerebrospinal fluid leak in posttraumatic and postsurgical patients.

INVESTIGATIONS (TYPICAL FINDINGS- BACTERIAL MENINGITIS)
- Lumbar puncture (LP) is the principal investigation (see Table 3.2) for example, in bacterial meningitis opening pressure is typically raised (20–40 cm H_2O) and cerebrospinal

fluid is cloudy, with a polymorphonuclear pleocytosis (100–10 000/mm^3). Bacteria may be visible on Gram stain. The polymerase chain reaction (PCR) is useful to detect bacterial antigens in partially treated meningitis. The protein level is elevated (100–500 mg/dL) and the glucose level is under 40% that of a simultaneously measured blood glucose.
- Peripheral white blood cells are increased with a left shift.
- *Blood and throat cultures:* To look for a source of infection and evidence of systemic sepsis.
- *Imaging:* CT and/or MRI is indicated to exclude the principal differential diagnoses of meningitis (subdural empyema, brain abscess and encephalitis) and to evaluate its complications.

Remember: LP must be preceded by a CT (or MRI) if there is any evidence of impairment of consciousness, focal neurological deficits or a prior seizure due to the risk of tonsillar herniation or coning.

MANAGEMENT
- Bacterial meningitis is a medical emergency and requires immediate antibiotic therapy. Broad-spectrum antibiotics are indicated while lumbar puncture results are awaited.
- *Neonate:* Ampicillin + third-generation cephalosporin or ampicillin + gentamicin.
- One–three months old: Ampicillin + third-generation cephalosporin.
- *Infant and child:* Ceftriaxone or cefotaxime.
- *Older child and adult:* Ceftriaxone or cefotaxime + ampicillin (if Listeria suspected).
- *More than 50 years old or alcoholic:* Third-generation cephalosporin + intravenous vancomycin.
- Change to specific antibiotics once culture results are available and continue antibiotics for 14 days.
- Dexamethasone reduces risk of deafness in children.

Remember: Meningitis is a medical emergency requiring urgent antibiotics, which should be commenced as soon as the disease is suspected, preferably after the CSF sample is obtained, provided this does not significantly delay treatment.

COMPLICATIONS   Arteritis, venous thrombosis, cerebral infarction; hydrocephalus; cranial nerve deficits; infected intracranial collections, including subdural empyema and cerebral abscess; ventriculitis; subdural effusions and seizure disorder.

PROGNOSIS   Neonatal meningitis carries a mortality of up to 50%. Of the survivors, 50% have permanent sequelae. *S. pneumoniae* and *N. meningitidis* meningitis carry a mortality of up to 25% and 10%, respectively.

DIFFERENTIAL DIAGNOSES (TABLE 21.1, ALSO SEE TABLE 4.2)

Table 21.1 Differential diagnoses with distinguishing features and points of note

Clinical conditions	How to exclude it
Viral meningitis	Enterovirus, mumps and Herpes simplex are the principal causes. Look for signs of systemic viraemia. Lumbar puncture: lymphocytic pleocytosis (<300/mm^3), normal glucose and normal to mildly elevated protein
TB meningitis	Consider other foci of tuberculous infection. Inflammation chronic, predominant in basal cisterns. Meningeal arteritis, cerebral infarction and hydrocephalus are frequent. Lumbar puncture: elevated opening pressure,

lymphocyte pleocytosis (100–500 cells/mm^3), elevated protein (100–200 mg/dL) and low glucose (<40 mg/dL). Cultures may not be positive for up to 8 weeks. PCR for tuberculous antigen may be useful

Fungal meningitis	*Cryptococcus*, *candida* and *Aspergillus* infections. Occur in immunocompromised hosts. Lumbar puncture findings as in TB meningitis. *C. neoformans* identified in India ink preparations of the cerebrospinal fluid, confirmed on positive latex agglutination test for cryptococcal polysaccharide antigen
Neoplastic meningitis	Associated with metastatic disease (leukaemia commonest in children; breast, lung and melanoma, in decreasing order, in adults). Lumbar puncture: elevated opening pressure, lymphocytic pleocytosis, low glucose and positive cytology for tumour in up to 80%. Postcontrast MRI shows leptomeningeal deposits, meningeal enhancement or hydrocephalus
Lyme disease	Meningoencephalitis, due to infection by *Borrelia burgdorferi*. Cranial or peripheral neuritis, particularly facial nerve involvement, erythema chronicum migrans, arthritis. Cerebrospinal fluid: lymphocytic pleocytosis (<3000/mm^3), elevated protein and normal glucose. Definitive diagnosis by lyme serology testing.
Encephalitis	Symptoms of meningitis are associated with impairment of consciousness, seizures and focal deficits. Cerebrospinal fluid: characterised by mononuclear pleocytosis, elevated protein, normal glucose and occasionally red cells, positive Herpes simplex virus PCR. Imaging (CT and MRI) shows asymmetric temporal lobe involvement in Herpes simplex encephalitis. EEG shows periodic high-voltage sharp waves and slow-wave complexes at 2–3 s intervals in the temporal leads
Subdural empyema	MRI demonstrates focal or diffuse subdural collection, with enhancing margins, cortical oedema and mass effect, often with evidence of cortical venous infarction. LP is not indicated and is potentially dangerous
Cerebral abscess (Chapter 22)	CT and MRI show ring-enhancing lesion with surrounding cerebral oedema and mass effect. May be multiple. Diffusion restricted on diffusion-weighted image. Lumbar puncture is potentially dangerous. Remember Toxoplasmosis is a potential agent causing cerebral abscess in an immunocompromised patient, for example with AIDS

Note on CSF shunt infections

- Meningitis/ventriculitis may follow insertion of a ventriculoperitoneal shunt, used to treat hydrocephalus. Infection may manifest in the postoperative period or in a delayed fashion weeks or even months later.
- Clinical features of meningitis may coexist with those of raised intracranial pressure due to associated shunt blockage. Urgent discussion with regional neurosurgical unit is advised as shunt is likely to require removal in addition to treatment of CSF infection.

22   Central nervous system infections: Cerebral abscess

DEFINITION   Encapsulated intraparenchymal necrotic infection characterised by a collection of pus.

EPIDEMIOLOGY   Risk factors as below. Current incidence approximately 2000 cases per year in the United States. Higher incidence in developing countries.

AETIOLOGY
- *Haematogenous spread (commonest cause of brain abscess):* Lung abscesses, bronchiectasis and pulmonary empyema; cyanotic congenital heart disease, particularly tetralogy of Fallot; pulmonary arteriovenous fistulas; acute bacterial endocarditis; dental infections; gastrointestinal infections and immunosuppression.
- *Contiguous spread:* Purulent sinusitis involving the middle ear, mastoid, nose or sphenoid sinuses.
- After neurosurgical procedure or penetrating cranial trauma.

> Remember: Haematogenous spread is the commonest cause of brain abscess.

PATHOLOGY/PATHOGENESIS   Streptococcus is the commonest organism. Multiple organisms are cultured in up to 30% of cases and usually include anaerobic, predominantly Bacteroides, species. The commonest posttraumatic and postneurosurgical organism is *Staphylococcus aureus*. *Toxoplasma* and *Nocardia* are likely organisms in immunocompromised patients.

There are four stages to the formation of a cerebral abscess, progressing from the early cerebritis phase, characterised by early focal parenchymal infection and infiltration, through late cerebritis (up to day 9, characterised by development of central necrosis) to capsule formation (early up to day 13 and late after day 14) with development of a collagen capsule, peri-capsular gliosis and a definite necrotic centre. The administration of corticosteroids tends to slow the progression.

HISTORY
- Symptoms suggestive of raised intracranial pressure, including headache, nausea and vomiting; irritability in children and seizures (may be focal or generalised and develop in up to 50% of cases).
- Development of a neurological deficit related to the abscess location; acute neurological deterioration may suggest intraventricular rupture of a brain abscess.
- Symptoms of primary infectious cause may be evident.

EXAMINATION
- Signs of elevated intracranial pressure, including impairment of consciousness, neck stiffness and focal neurological deficit.
- Evidence of primary infection, for example lung or sinuses.
- May not necessarily be associated with pyrexia.

INVESTIGATIONS
- Peripheral white cell count, erythrocyte sedimentation rate and blood cultures—often within normal limits or negative.
- C-reactive protein may be elevated in relation to the primary or systemic infection.
- Imaging is the investigative modality of choice. CT with contrast can be used to demonstrate ring enhancement (Figure 22.1). A mature encapsulated abscess shows ring enhancement of the capsule on postcontrast MRI. Extensive pericapsular oedema is

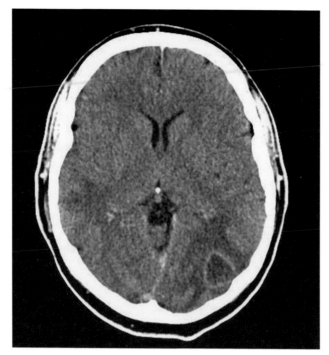

Figure 22.1 CT demonstrates a left occipital abscess with associated hypodensity (oedema) and enhancement with contrast.

evident. The necrotic centre demonstrates restricted diffusion on diffusion-weighted imaging. In the early cerebritis phase, the lesion is hypointense and hyperintense on T1- and T2-weighted images, respectively. Magnetic resonance spectroscopy shows high lactate, alanine and glycine in the necrotic centre of a mature abscess, while *N*-acetyl aspartate, creatine and choline peaks are reduced (compare with choline peaks in malignant glioma) (Table 22.1).

- *Other investigations directed at finding the source of abscess:* Echocardiogram, CT of chest and abdomen, orthopantomogram (dental X-ray), CT of sinuses and so on.

> *Remember: Investigations directed towards detecting underlying source of abscess are important for treating the source and preventing future recurrence.*

MANAGEMENT

- Surgical drainage, usually by needle aspiration under image guidance, or excision of the abscess if superficially located in non-eloquent brain is the primary treatment. This is indicated to reduce the mass effect exerted by an abscess; obtain an organism to guide antimicrobial therapy and get a definitive diagnosis of an abscess if imaging is uncertain and to reduce the risk of intraventricular rupture when the abscess is close to the ventricular wall. Multiple small abscesses may not be amenable to surgical drainage and may be best managed medically.

- Medical management is critical and includes appropriate antimicrobial therapy, initially broad-spectrum, intravenous (often including vancomycin, third-generation cephalosporin and metronidazole) and subsequently tailored to isolated organism and its sensitivity; corticosteroids to reduce oedema associated with the abscess and to control its mass effect (should only be used in conjunction with antibiotics); and diuretics to control elevated intracranial pressure if necessary. The recommended duration of antibiotics is generally 6–8 weeks, depending on confirmation of falling C-reactive protein levels and reduction in abscess size on serial imaging.

COMPLICATIONS   *Intraventricular rupture with ventriculitis* (often fatal); seizure disorder and focal neurological deficit.

PROGNOSIS   Current mortality is approximately 10% with a worse prognosis associated with poor neurological function, intraventricular rupture and fungal abscesses in transplant recipients.

DIFFERENTIAL DIAGNOSES

Table 22.1 Differential diagnoses/related conditions with distinguishing features

Clinical conditions	How to exclude it
Subdural empyema	Purulent infection of the subdural space, usually related to sinus, ear or mastoid infection; best visualised on postcontrast MRI, with oedema of the underlying hemisphere. Urgent craniotomy and evacuation is indicated
Extradural abscess	Purulent collection in the extradural space, usually frontal and related to frontal sinus infection; associated with local tenderness, subcutaneous swelling and erythema. Postcontrast MRI demonstrates an enhancing lenticular collection; local osteomyelitis may be evident on a CT scan. Urgent evacuation is indicated
Malignant glial tumour (Chapter 36)	May also demonstrate ring enhancement and a necrotic centre on imaging; tumour wall usually more irregular than abscess capsule. Magnetic resonance spectroscopy shows high lactate and choline (compare with abscess); free diffusion on diffusion-weighted MR (compare with abscess). Surgical needle aspiration is indicated if unable to clearly differentiate between two diagnoses on MRI
Metastatic tumour (Chapter 36)	As above—may also demonstrate necrotic centre and smooth wall and be difficult to differentiate from abscess radiologically. In the absence of multiple systemic lesions or a known primary tumour, needle aspiration of the brain lesion may be necessary
Toxoplasmosis	Occurs in immunocompromised patients, particularly those with AIDS. Demonstrated on imaging as a multifocal encephalitis with inflammatory necrotic foci; diagnosis established by elevation of serologic titres. Organism not usually found in the CSF. Brain biopsy may be required to differentiate from lymphoma in AIDS patients. Needs treatment with pyrimethamine and sulphadiazine
Nocardia	Bacterial infection occurring in immunocompromised patients. Haematogenous spread; brain involvement usually associated with peripheral soft tissue abscesses. May require brain biopsy if isolated. Needs trimethoprim–sulphamethoxazole in combination with cephalosporin

23   Radiculopathy and disc herniation   *LMN*

DEFINITION   Radiculopathy refers to a disease process affecting the nerve roots leading to pain in the distribution of the nerve root, dermatomal sensory disturbance with weakness of muscles supplied by the nerve root and suppressed or absent relevant reflexes. The primary focus in this chapter will be on spinal disc herniation.

AETIOLOGY   The commonest cause is compression by a prolapsed intervertebral disc (acute disc) in the cervical (usually C5/C6 or C6/C7 level) or lumbar spine (usually L4/L5 or L5/S1 level) usually in younger patients. Nucleus pulposus herniates through the ruptured annulus fibrosus. Other causes include degenerative cervical or lumbar spondylotic disease in the elderly population with rarer causes being tumours both benign, i.e. schwannomas and meningiomas, and malignant (compression from bony metastasis); inflammatory (Herpes virus infection and shingles) and malignant meningitis.

ASSOCIATIONS/RISK FACTORS   Depends upon the cause. With lumbar and cervical discs, there may be a recent history of heavy lifting or straining.

PATHOLOGY/PATHOGENESIS   See above. Lumbar discs usually herniate posterolaterally causing nerve root compression, as posterior longitudinal ligament is strongest in the midline. When the ruptured disc is large and midline, cauda equina syndrome (CES) may result.

HISTORY

Lumbar discs: Back pain (usually minor component of history); radicular pain (known as sciatica when referring to L5 and S1 roots due to distribution along sciatic nerve) radiating into legs, terminating in dermatome of compressed root; avoidance of movements; weakness and sensory disturbance in nerve root distribution; sphincter disturbance (bowel and bladder symptoms) (see CES).

Cervical discs: Lead to limitation of neck movement with radicular pain (known as 'brachialgia') radiating from neck into the shoulders and arms with or without motor and/or sensory symptoms.

EXAMINATION

Lumbosacral spine: Lasegue's sign or straight leg raise test involves raising the affected limb by ankle until patient complains of pain radiating down the leg below the knee, exacerbated by ankle dorsiflexion. When positive, pain occurs at <60 degrees as the test leads to tensing of L5 and S1 primarily and to a smaller extent the more proximal roots. A positive femoral stretch test (hip extension followed by knee flexion, causing anterior thigh pain) is positive with L2, L3 or L4 nerve root compression. With L5/S1 prolapse (about 50% of cases) involving S1, root findings may be weakness in plantarflexion (ask patient to stand on tiptoes one leg at a time) and depressed ankle jerk with reduction of sensation in lateral aspect and the sole of foot (S1 distribution). An L4/L5 disc prolapse impinging upon L5 root may cause weakness of dorsiflexion or foot drop (ask patient to walk on their heels); extensor hallucis longus weakness and sensory loss in dorsum of foot.

Remember: In lumbar spine, a herniated lumbar disc usually compresses the nerve root exiting from the foramen below the level of herniation; therefore, an L5/S1 disc prolapse will impinge upon the 'transiting' S1 root, as it passes through the lateral recess of the spinal canal before it exits below the pedicle of its corresponding vertebra.

Cervical spine: A C6/C7 disc prolapse compressing C7 root may cause diminished triceps reflex; weakness of triceps with sensory symptoms in C7 distribution. A C5/C6 disc impinging upon C6 root may cause diminished biceps reflex with weakness in biceps (forearm flexion) and sensory symptoms in C6 distribution.

Remember: In cervical spine, a herniated disc compresses on the nerve root exiting from the foramen at the level of the herniation as the nerve root exits above the pedicle of its corresponding vertebra (refer to lumbar spine); therefore, a C6/C7 prolapse impinges upon C7 root. The exception is the C8 root which exits below the C7 pedicle at the C7/ T1 level.

INVESTIGATIONS

Lumbosacral spine: Majority with disc herniation improve spontaneously (up to 70% within 4 weeks). In the absence of red flag signs (see below), no imaging tests are required in the first 4 weeks. The recommended tests include standing AP and lateral view of the spine to assess for scoliosis or other spinal deformity and spondylolisthesis (a forward 'slip' of one vertebrae on the vertebrae below due to a defect in the pars interarticularis); MRI (currently the test of choice) (Figure 23.1); CT and myelography

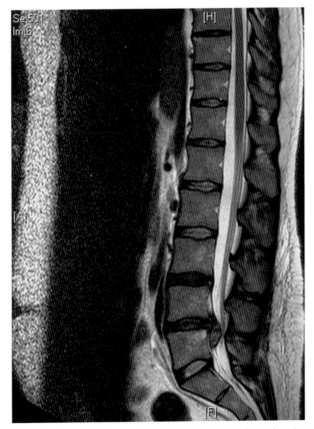

Figure 23.1 MRI of lumbosacral spine demonstrating disc prolapse at L4/L5 causing cauda equina syndrome.

(when MRI cannot be done). As a guide, obtain imaging when either red flag signs are present (e.g. indicating CES) or symptoms of prolapsed disc severe enough to consider surgery persist beyond 4 weeks. Blood tests (FBC and ESR) should be performed with suspected infection or malignancy.

Cervical spine: MRI of the cervical spine is the study of choice. Consider plain CT and myelogram if MRI is contraindicated or better bony detail is required.

MANAGEMENT

Lumbosacral spine: Majority with herniated lumbar discs improve without surgery (conservative treatment with analgesia and reduction in heavy exercises) over an average period of 6 weeks. Prolonged bed rest is not necessary. Consider surgery if symptoms persist beyond 5–8 weeks. Emergent surgery is indicated in the presence of CES, progressive weakness, for example foot drop, or severe unremitting pain despite adequate analgesia. Surgical options include lumbar microdiscectomy or laminectomy and discectomy for very large disc prolapses.

Cervical Spine: Majority with herniated cervical discs improve without surgery. Analgesics as necessary. Consider surgery (anterior cervical discectomy with fusion or cervical arthroplasty; posterior foraminotomy) if conservative treatment fails or progressive neurological deficits develop.

COMPLICATIONS

Cauda equina syndrome: CES usually develops due to a large central ruptured disc compressing the cauda equina and can present acutely or slowly. Other causes include malignant compression or a spinal extradural haematoma from trauma. Important symptoms and signs may be low back pain with bilateral sciatica, saddle anaesthesia (in the region of anus, perineum and buttocks), progressive lower extremity weakness, bilateral absent ankle reflexes and disturbances of sphincter function including urinary retention and urinary and/or faecal incontinence with or without reduction in anal tone on digital rectal examination. Surgery to remove disc should be performed within 48 h of onset of CES symptoms, preferably within 24 h if possible.

> *Remember:* CES must be suspected in patients presenting with low back pain, sciatica and sphincter disturbance. A full neurological examination including testing of anal tone and perineal sensation is mandatory with an MRI of lumbosacral spine if appropriate to exclude this pathology. Emergent decompression (laminectomy and discectomy) is advised. Missing this pathology has enormous medicolegal implications.

Note on Red Flag Signs for Imaging

In a patient with low back pain and sciatica, a serious condition, for example infection, malignancy or CES should be considered in the presence of the following signs and symptoms and urgent MR imaging should be undertaken and the case discussed with a neurosurgeon. Other investigations such as CT or plain X-rays may be appropriate. Suggestive of CES: as above; suggestive of spinal fracture: history of trauma, elderly osteoporotic patient (e.g. on long-term steroids) and thoracic pain; suggestive of malignancy: age >55 or <20 years, recent weight loss or previous history of cancer, unrelenting pain at rest, pain waking from sleep at night (recumbent pain) and thoracic pain; suggestive of infection (discitis or epidural abscess): temperature, alcoholic or IVDU, diabetics, immunosuppressed patients, recent spinal surgery or infection, for example UTI.

> *Remember: Always treat recumbent back pain suspiciously as it may denote malignancy.*

24 Peripheral neuropathies' syndromes

DEFINITION/INTRODUCTION   Disorders of peripheral nerves may involve a single nerve (mononeuropathy), multiple single nerves (multiple mononeuropathy/mononeuritis multiplex) or a generalised dysfunction of peripheral nerves (polyneuropathy). The pathway of a peripheral nerve may be compromised at various points along its course: cell body, nerve root, plexus (brachial/lumbosacral), axon, myelin sheath or nerve terminal. Alternatively, the entire length of the nerve may degenerate (neuronopathy). Different types of peripheral nerves may be variably affected (e.g. isolated motor, sensory or autonomic nerve dysfunction or a combination of all three). Likewise, different anatomical fibre types may be variously affected: large fibre, small fibre, myelinated or unmyelinated nerve fibres.

Peripheral nerve disorders may arise due to primary (genetic) or secondary (acquired) causes. Particular causative diseases often have a predilection for specific nerve or fibre types and for certain components of the nerve course. For example, diabetic neuropathy most commonly affects the axons of small-diameter sensory nerves in a length-dependent manner (i.e. longest nerves damaged first and most affected), hence these patients typically report a symmetrical sensory disturbance of the feet producing numbness and pain in a stocking distribution.

Peripheral nerve disorders may be acute (reaching maximum severity before 4 weeks), subacute (reaching maximum severity between 4 and 8 weeks) or chronically progressive (taking more than 8 weeks to reach maximum severity). Peripheral nerve symptoms may present with additional associated features, for example pain associated with the sensory disturbance of diabetic neuropathy.

A careful and full history and examination often allows determination of the type of underlying process (single nerve, multiple nerves and generalised), the portion of the nerve or nerves involved and the causation.

EPIDEMIOLOGY   Common, for example the prevalence of a symmetrical, length-dependent, sensory, axonal, polyneuropathy producing numbness of the feet occurs in approximately 2% of the elderly. Mononeuropathies are also very common, for example carpal tunnel syndrome (CTS) due to entrapment of the median nerve at the wrist occurs in 5% of women.

HISTORY   Elicit following from the history:
- Ascertain body region or regions where symptoms are experienced, including their distribution—Does this match with a specific nerve root or roots, specific nerve or nerves? Are the symptoms suggestive of a more generalised nerve dysfunction?
- When did the symptoms start and can a triggering cause be identified?
- Are the symptoms continuous or episodic? If episodic, what are the provoking and relieving factors and how often and for how long do the symptoms occur?
- What is the temporal course? Did symptoms progress to reach maximum within days to weeks or is there continuing deterioration?
- Check the past medical history for disorders causing neuropathy as an associated feature (e.g. vitamin B12 deficiency).
- A developmental history looking for long-standing problems arising in childhood, such as difficulty with school sports, may be seen in genetic causes of polyneuropathy which produces long-standing symptoms.
- Medication history as many cause neuropathy as a side effect.
- Family history in cases of genetic/inherited forms of neuropathy (in the earlier generations, symptoms and signs may be absent or mild, for example a history of high arched feet).
- *Social history*: Check for alcohol consumption and illicit drug use. Alcohol overuse is one of the commonest causes of a symmetrical sensory polyneuropathy (numb feet with

absent ankle jerks) but may also produce isolated failure of single nerves, for example a radial nerve palsy leading to wrist drop.

- A systems' review to identify problems outside the peripheral nerves associated with neuropathy (e.g. lung cancer leading to a rapidly progressive polyneuropathy as a para-neoplastic phenomenon).

Remember: Alcohol overuse is one of the commonest causes of a symmetrical sensory polyneuropathy.

EXAMINATION   In addition to a full neurological examination with particular attention to absent reflexes, the following points should be considered:

- Look for muscle wasting documenting whether the distribution is distal (hands and feet) or proximal (hips and shoulders) and symmetrical or asymmetrical.
- Look for fasciculation, indicating a lower motor neurone problem, often indicating damage/degeneration of the cell body (anterior horn cell).
- Look for pes cavus and claw toes; evidence that peripheral neuropathy has been present since early childhood and produced developmental deformity.
- Look for associated skin and nail changes. These may be seen in, for example, diabetes or a vasculitic process which may produce a multiple mononeuropathy.
- Palpate nerves to look for evidence of thickening as can be seen in leprosy.
- Detail the pattern of weakness noting whether it is distal or proximal and symmetrical or asymmetrical.
- Reflex testing is crucial. However, note that patients often have types of peripheral nerve dysfunction not causing a loss of reflexes (e.g. most times in mononeuropathy or multi-ple mononeuropathy and in polyneuropathy of a small fibre type).
- Sensory testing should include various modalities to contrast different fibre types and pathways, for example pinprick sensation versus proprioception and vibration sense.
- Draw out areas of reduced sensation to determine if this maps to a single root (derma-tome) or single nerve, for example sensory disturbance in the medial portion of the palm and in the little and medial half of the ring finger in case of ulnar nerve entrapment at the elbow.

INVESTIGATIONS   Nerve conduction studies (NCS) help differentiate whether a single nerve is involved or multiple single nerves or a more generalised polyneuropathy. Similarly, whether the problem is exclusively in sensory nerves, motor nerves or a combination can be determined. By assessing the velocity of conduction and amplitude of conduction, it can be understood if the axon or the myelin sheath is predominantly affected.

Remember: In general, conduction velocity falls with demyelination whereas the ampli-tude decreases with axonal dysfunction/degeneration.

Extensive blood testing: To look for causes of secondary generalised polyneuropathies particularly as identifying such causes may result in reversal of symptoms or at least halt-ing of progression. A typical screen (depending on the history and examination) includes glucose, FBC, B12, U & E, LFT, Ca, TFT, CRP, PV, autoimmune profile, ACE, immunoglo-bilins, serum electrophoresis and urine for Bence Jones protein. In addition, infections may be looked for, including HIV, syphilis, lyme, chronic hepatitis and in cases of suspected paraneoplastic process test for paraneoplastic antibodies.

Lumbar puncture is helpful in specific situations, for example, in demyelinating neuropa-thies like Guillian–Barré syndrome (GBS) or chronic inflammatory demyelinating polyneuropathy (CIDP), where a raised CSF protein is typically seen (see later).

MANAGEMENT   Identifying the cause is the most important management step as it may allow cure or a halting or limiting of progression (e.g. managing diabetes more closely in diabetic neuropathy; reducing alcohol intake in an alcohol-induced neuropathy; median nerve decompression in CTS or treating GBS with intravenous immunoglobulin (IVIG)).

If irreversible or a cause is not identified, generic symptomatic treatments are employed to reduce neuropathy-related discomfort and pain such as amitriptyline or certain anticonvulsant medications.

A multidisciplinary team (MDT) approach to optimise aspects such as foot care and walking aids and treatment of autonomic dysfunction is also important.

DIFFERENTIAL DIAGNOSES   It is important to consider that the sensory disturbance, motor weakness or autonomic failure observed may not be due to a peripheral nerve disorder but rather due to a central problem (brain/spinal cord) or in some cases due to isolated weakness related to disturbance of neuromuscular junction, for example Myasthenia gravis or in some other cases due to isolated muscle pathology, for example myositis.

Guillain–Barré syndrome

DEFINITION   It is an acute inflammatory demyelinating polyradiculoneuropathy. In approximately 10% of patients, however, the acute neuropathy is axonal rather than demyelinating. It is typically a monophasic, predominantly motor polyradiculopathy. By definition, such acute polyneuropathies reach maximal severity within 4 weeks.

EPIDEMIOLOGY   GBS is more common in the elderly, although it occurs at any age and in both males and females. GBS is the commonest cause of an acute peripheral paralysis.

AETIOLOGY   Close to two-thirds of patients have had an infection during the preceding 6 weeks. Most often this is a respiratory tract infection but if gastrointestinal, *Campylobacter jejuni* is the commonest cause.

PATHOLOGY/PATHOGENESIS   GBS is an autoimmune disease triggered by preceding infection.

HISTORY   Pain in the lower back is often the first symptom. Initial weakness may be proximal, distal or both and may progress in either a descending or ascending fashion. Sensory disturbance is common. The face and bulbar muscles are often affected.

EXAMINATION
- Tone may be normal or reduced.
- Reflexes are characteristically lost but may remain present early in the condition.
- Sensory testing must be performed.
- Autonomic disturbance must be looked for and monitored (pulse, blood pressure and heart rhythm) as arrhythmias and hypotension or hypertension may result. The autonomic nervous system is affected to varying extent in this condition.

INVESTIGATIONS
- Nerve conduction studies may be normal during the first few days but then demonstrate slowing of motor nerve conduction and partial conduction block in the demyelinating form of GBS or reduction in compound muscle action potentials with preserved conduction velocity in the axonal form of GBS.
- CSF often shows an increased protein level but may be normal early on. The white cell count is normal or only minimally raised <10, i.e. the so-called *albuminocytologic dissociation* is usually observed.
- IgG antibodies to ganglioside GM1 are present in a quarter of patients, more often in those with acute motor axonal neuropathy.
- It is important to consider the other differentials for an acute polyradiculoneuropathy, including infective, toxic, metabolic or vasculitic causes.

MANAGEMENT   First consider life-threatening complications: measure vital capacity and assess bulbar function, monitor heart rhythm for arrhythmias, blood pressure for sudden surges or falls and administer DVT/PE prophylaxis.

IVIG is the mainstay of treatment. An alternative is plasma exchange; steroids are not helpful.

Ventilatory support in the intensive care unit may be required along with management of any autonomic disturbance.

> *Remember: Regular measurement of vital capacity in these patients is very important as those with a VC < 1 L may require ventilation.*

Note on Chronic Inflammatory Demyelinating Polyneuropathy (CIDP)

CIDP shares some similarities with GBS but in contrast is not an acute condition but rather is chronic in its course and is typically relapsing. The first presentation develops over more than 8 weeks. Differentiating CIDP from a chronic axonal neuropathy is important because CIDP responds to therapy. The diagnosis requires nerve conduction studies demonstrating conduction slowing. The mainstay of treatment is immune suppression and in contrast to GBS, steroids are helpful.

25 Common peripheral nerve lesions: Mononeuropathies

DEFINITION   Individual peripheral nerves can be damaged as a result of trauma, compression or entrapment of the nerve. Any peripheral nerve can be damaged; however, some nerves are more susceptible to damage than others due to their more exposed anatomical position, especially as they pass along bones and through fibrous arches. In the upper limb, the median, ulnar and radial nerves are most commonly damaged; in the lower limb, the common peroneal nerve is most often damaged.

EPIDEMIOLOGY   Mononeuropathies can affect anyone. Factors that make nerves more susceptible to damage are trauma/pressure, diabetes, thyroid dysfunction, vitamin deficiencies, alcoholism, certain infections, autoimmune diseases, tumour, inherited disorders and some genes.

Carpal tunnel syndrome (CTS) is the commonest form of nerve entrapment (median nerve) and is more common in women than men with a mean age of onset between 30 and 40 years. Common peroneal neuropathies are almost three times more common in men than women.

Mononeuropathies tend to be unilateral; however, approximately 60% of patients with CTS present with bilateral symptoms, normally with more severe symptoms in the dominant hand. About 10% of common peroneal neuropathies are also bilateral.

AETIOLOGY
Median nerve palsy:
Common site of damage: Carpal tunnel.
- *CTS:* Compression of the median nerve as it runs through the carpal tunnel; most common cause.
- *Trauma:* Wrist lacerations.

Ulnar nerve palsy:
Common sites of damage:
(1)   Behind the medial epicondyle of the humerus and in the cubital tunnel.
- *Compression.* Repetitive application of external pressure:
  ○   Resting elbow on a firm surface (a desk or the base of a car window frame).
  ○   Malpositioning/inadequate padding during surgery or while in a coma.
- *Elbow deformities.* Congenital anomalies, osteoarthritis and rheumatoid arthritis.
(2)   In the wrist and hand.
- *Trauma.* Wrist lacerations, puncture wounds to hand (industrial accidents).
- Compression by external pressure (cycling, use of a cane or volleyball).

Radial nerve palsy:
Common site of damage: Spiral groove of humerus.
- *Trauma:* The commonest traumatic cause is fracture of the humerus.
- Compression against the lateral aspect of the arm:
  ○   Patients lying on their arm for a prolonged time.
  ○   Tourniquet paralysis.

Common peroneal nerve palsy:
Common site of damage: As it winds around the head of the fibula.
- *Compression*
  ○   Prolonged squatting (strawberry pickers, palsy).
  ○   Exposure to pressure (e.g. leg crossing) after weight loss and therefore loss of subcutaneous fat padding.
  ○   Malpositioning/inadequate padding during surgery or while in a coma.
- *Trauma:* Fibular fractures, knee dislocation, dislocation of the superior tibiofibular joint, ligament ruptures of the knee joint and animal bites.

In addition to the above causes, any nerve palsy can also result from blunt trauma such as lacerations (from knives or glass), gunshot wounds and space-occupying lesions (neural sheath tumours, primary nerve tumours, lipomas and ganglion cysts).

PATHOLOGY/PATHOGENESIS   Compression injury leads to demyelinating conduction block; trauma leads to axon loss with recovery dependent on reinnervation.

HISTORY/EXAMINATION   This is summarised in Table 25.1 detailing common named nerve palsies.

Special tests:
- *Tinel's sign:* Gentle percussion of the affected nerves reproduce numbness and tingling in patients with median, ulnar and common peroneal nerve palsies.
- The numbness, tingling or pain experienced by patients with CTS can be reproduced by extreme flexion of the wrist for 1 min (Phalen's manoeuvre) and by holding the affected hand over the head for 2 min.

Table 25.1 Common named nerve palsies with symptoms and signs

	Sensory symptoms	Motor symptoms	Signs
Median nerve palsy	Numbness, tingling and pain (less common); can get symptoms in ulnar fingers	Thenar muscle weakness, especially abductor pollicis brevis: inability to oppose the thumb and difficulty in gripping/holding objects (e.g. difficulty in buttoning up shirts)	Patients may have impaired two-point discrimination or pain perception; thenar muscle weakness and atrophy
Ulnar nerve palsy	Tingling and possibly pain (Figure 25.1)	Weakness of medial wrist flexors and the intrinsic muscles of the hand; *claw hand* (extended MCP and flexed interphalangeal joints), more marked in wrist lesion	Muscle weakness and atrophy (in severe cases). If the lesion occurs at the elbow, the nerve may be enlarged and tender on palpation and elbow flexion can precipitate or exaggerate symptoms
Radial nerve palsy	Loss of sensation over dorsum of hand (Figure 25.2)	Wrist drop and finger drop: weakness in extensors of the wrist and metacarpophalangeal joints; can get weakness in the triceps—flexed elbow	Loss of reflexes: supinator and triceps (if the lesion is in or near the axilla); muscle weakness
Common peroneal palsy	Numbness over dorsum of foot, can extend into the lower lateral leg and in proximal lesions to the upper lateral leg and knee; can be accompanied by mild deep, boring pain	Complete or partial *foot drop*: weakness of the tibialis anterior and other extensors of the foot and toes; may lead to repeated falls, foot or ankle sprains and fractures	Weak ankle and toe dorsiflexion and ankle eversion; impaired touch and pain sensation over the lower 2/3 of the lateral leg and the dorsum of the foot

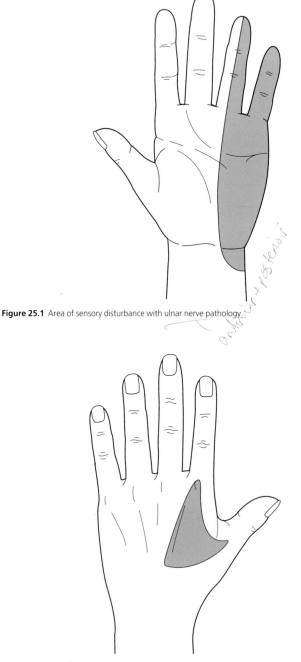

Figure 25.1 Area of sensory disturbance with ulnar nerve pathology.

anterior + posterior

Figure 25.2 Area of sensory disturbance with radial nerve pathology.

Remember to memorise Table 25.1 *well with named nerve palsies as commonly tested in exams.*

INVESTIGATIONS AND DIAGNOSIS   Mainly based on history and clinical examination (especially muscle weakness as sensation testing can be unreliable). Physical examination (Table 25.1) is also important to exclude any other neurological conditions, upper motor neuron lesions and the involvement of other nerves or nerve roots.

Nerve conduction studies, electromyography, ultrasound scans, neuroimaging and radio-imaging can also aid the diagnosis.

MANAGEMENT

Demyelinating conduction block: Patients normally recover fully with conservative treatments, for example splint, especially at night, change in work environment to minimise further pressure, padding and anti-inflammatories (steroids). Some recover spontaneously without any treatment.

Axon loss: Patients tend to require surgical treatment, except radial nerve damage as a result of fractured humerus where conservative treatment is normally sufficient. Recovery can be slow and in some cases incomplete depending on the location and severity of nerve damage.

In CTS there may be an underlying cause of the nerve entrapment, which may require surgical treatment.

26   Motor neurone disease (MND)

DEFINITION   Also known as amyotrophic (muscle wasting) lateral (corticospinal tracts) sclerosis (scarring) (ALS) or Lou Gehrig's disease in the United States. A progressive disorder characterised by degeneration of motor neurones of the central and peripheral nervous system, thereby producing UMN or LMN signs or most commonly a combination of both with sparing of the sensory and autonomic system. MND comprises several syndromes:

- *Progressive bulbar palsy (PBP):* LMN bulbar symptoms and signs predominate.
- *Classical Charcot ALS:* The commonest form, mixed upper and lower motor neurone signs.
- *Primary lateral sclerosis (PLS):* Isolated UMN signs due to degeneration of corticospinal tracts.
- *Progressive muscular atrophy (PMA):* Isolated LMN signs due to degeneration of anterior horn cells.

Remember: Although the different syndromes in MND progress with a varying rate of evolution, eventually they overlap significantly and in late stages merge into a diffuse combined UMN and LMN disorder.

EPIDEMIOLOGY
- *Incidence:* Approximately 1–3 per 100 000 per year.
- *Mean age at the onset:* 60 years (male:female ratio = 1.7:1).
- *Main risk factors:* Increasing age, gender and family history.
- Twenty-five per cent of MND patients present with PBP.

AETIOLOGY
- *Sporadic*:
  - Most cases; unknown aetiology.
  - Toxic role for the excitatory amino acid neurotransmitter glutamate suggested.
- *Genetic*:
  - Family history seen in 5–10%.
  - Some rare families show autosomal dominant transmission.
  - In almost 20% of familial cases, a mutation on chromosome 21 in the gene encoding the free radical scavenging enzyme copper/zinc superoxide dismutase (SOD1) is seen (exactly how this produces motor neurone degeneration is unknown, but potentially oxidative injury occurs as a result of increased free radical production).

ASSOCIATIONS/RISK FACTORS   See section 'Epidemiology'.

PATHOLOGY/PATHOGENESIS
- Degeneration of pyramidal cells within the motor cortex and corticospinal tracts produce UMN signs.
- Degeneration of large anterior horn cells in the spinal cord and brainstem motor nuclei produce LMN signs.

HISTORY   Onset typically occurs in the following:
- One arm leading to weakness of grip.
- One leg causing foot drop.
- Followed by generalisation of the symptoms with eventual involvement of truncal and bulbar muscles.

PBP
- Common in older women.

- Related to degeneration of lower motor nerves in the brainstem (bulb).
- Usually presents with dysarthria and dysphagia (wasted, fasciculating tongue and wasted pharyngeal muscles).
- Often combined with a pseudo-bulbar syndrome (UMN-type syndrome with emotional lability; stiff tongue; spastic dysarthria; brisk facial, snout and jaw jerk reflexes and nasality).
- Limb involvement usually follows within months.

EXAMINATION
- Demonstrates combined UMN (spastic tonal increase, pyramidal pattern weakness, pathologically brisk reflexes and upgoing plantars) and LMN (wasting, fasciculation, weakness and reflex loss) signs in various affected regions.
- Careful examination reveals the absence of visual, sensory or cerebellar signs.

Remember: The combination of UMN and LMN signs differentiates this condition from many others affecting the motor system. The sensory and autonomic nervous system (bladder and bowel) is spared along with motor neurones controlling eye movements (extraocular muscles).

INVESTIGATIONS
- No single diagnostic test for MND.
- *Blood:* To rule out other conditions (Table 26.1).
- *EMG:* Confirms LMN loss by showing denervation, fasciculations, fibrillation and giant motor unit potentials (MUPs).
- *Normal nerve conduction study:* Confirms absence of sensory abnormality and absence of motor neurone axonopathy/demyelination to account for LMN signs.
- *MRI of spine and brain:* Excludes other abnormalities.

Remember: Diagnosis relies on careful clinical examination and exclusion of other differentials (Table 26.1).

MANAGEMENT
- *Medical*
  - Riluzole, an antiglutamate agent (promoted as slowing disease progression): Only a modest effect in prolonging survival with an increase in life expectancy by 2–4 months at 18 months.
  - Riluzole is prescribed early in the disease and requires regular monitoring of liver function tests (can lead to deranged liver enzymes).

Other medications to improve symptoms include antispasticity agents like baclofen or tizanidine and antidepressants for mood disorders.
- *Supportive*
  - A multidisciplinary team of physiotherapists, occupational therapists, speech and language therapists, dieticians and MND nurses are required to deliver good care.
  - Percutaneous endoscopic gastrostomy and non-invasive pressure ventilation may be required to combat swallowing and ventilatory difficulties as the disease progresses.

Remember: There is no cure for MND and Riluzole is the only drug with a proven benefit in patients' survival.

COMPLICATIONS   Progressive loss of mobility, ability to speak, swallowing (weight loss and aspiration pneumonia) and subsequently respiratory difficulties leading to death.

PROGNOSIS   Death occurs most commonly due to respiratory failure or concurrent infection with the mean survival from the onset of symptoms being 3 years. Prognosis is worse for elderly, female or bulbar onset patients.

DIFFERENTIAL DIAGNOSES

Table 26.1 Differential diagnoses with appropriate investigations

Clinical conditions	How to exclude it (investigations to do)
Degenerative spinal cord disease leading to myeloradiculopathy (Chapter 23)	MRI scan of the spinal cord (may be reversed or halted with neurosurgery)
Multifocal motor neuropathy with conduction block; other polyneuropathies or mononeuritis multiplex	EMG, NCS and antiganglioside Ab (may be reversed or halted with immune therapies such as intravenous gamma globulin)
Spinal muscular atrophy and Kennedy's disease	Genetic studies
Thyrotoxicosis causing bulbar muscle or proximal weakness	Thyroid function tests
Diabetic amyotrophy, i.e. muscle wasting	Blood glucose, HbA1c and EMG
Inflammatory myopathies (Chapter 28)	Measure CK (only mildly raised in MND)

27   Myasthenia gravis and Lambert–Eaton myasthenic syndrome

DEFINITION   Myasthenia gravis (MG) is an autoimmune disease characterised by the presence of autoantibodies directed against postsynaptic acetylcholine (Ach) receptors at the neuromuscular junction (NMJ).

EPIDEMIOLOGY
- Male:female ratio of MG in children and adults is 2:3 with a female predominance in younger age group (20–30 years) and a mild male predominance in older patients (>50 years old).
- MG can occur at any age.

AETIOLOGY   Uncertain.

ASSOCIATIONS/RISK FACTORS
- Association with other autoimmune disorders, including thyroid disease and thymus gland disorders, for example thymoma or thymic hyperplasia.
- In younger patients, MG is associated with thymic hyperplasia and other autoimmune conditions; in older patients (>50 years), MG is associated with thymic atrophy or tumour.
- Drugs, including beta-blockers, calcium channel blockers, sedatives, D-penicillamine, aminoglycoside antibiotics (gentamicin), neuromuscular blockers (succinylcholine and vecuronium) may all aggravate MG and lead to a myasthenic crisis.

> Remember the association between MG and thymus gland disorders.

PATHOLOGY/PATHOGENESIS
- MG is mediated by antibodies (IgG) directed against the acetylcholine receptor (AchR) found on the *postsynaptic* membrane at the NMJ.
- This decreases the number of functional AchRs resulting in impaired neuromuscular transmission.

HISTORY
- Symptoms may have been present for months or years.
- Cardinal feature is variable weakness and fatigue of voluntary muscles (fatiguability) with diurnal variation, which may be evident with symptoms worsening towards the end of the day.
- Patients may report episodic double vision and droopy eyelids (ptosis) with possible weakness of eye closure, facial weakness, problems with speech and swallowing, breathing difficulties, neck weakness and proximal limb weakness (relative sparing of lower limbs).
- Patients can present with sudden myasthenic crisis.

> Remember: Variable muscle weakness and fatiguability of voluntary muscles in MG. Persistent ocular involvement (ocular myasthenia) occurs in less than 20% as about 80% of patients go on to develop generalised MG within a year of the onset of symptom.

EXAMINATION
- Usually tone, reflexes and sensation are normal.
- Weakness may be evident or power may be normal in which case clinical tests for fatiguability should be performed.

- o *Eyes*: Ask the patient to sustain upgaze for 30 s—ptosis or diplopia may be provoked.
- o *Speech (bulbar)*: For example, ask the patient to count up to 50.
- *Arms (proximal muscle)*: Ask the patient to perform repeated shoulder abduction (20–30 times) and assess shoulder abduction strength before and after.
- Examination may demonstrate ptosis, diplopia and the characteristic myasthenic snarl on smiling.
- Muscle groups involved in decreasing order of frequency are extraocular, bulbar, face, neck, proximal limbs and trunk.

INVESTIGATIONS
- *Blood tests*: AchR antibodies are present (sero-positive) in up to 90% of patients with generalised MG.
- *Neurophysiology*:
  - o *Decrement* of compound muscle action potentials (cMAPs) on repetitive stimulation (proximal muscle).
  - o Presence of increased jitter on single-fibre EMG.
- *Intravenous edrophonium (short acting cholinesterase inhibitor) test*:
  - o Resuscitation facilities must be available when carrying out this test.
  - o Administer covering dose of atropine prior to giving Edrophonium.
  - o The positive effect (evident within a few seconds and lasting for a few minutes only) can be assessed using ptosis, diplopia or limb strength as a measure.
  - o The risks are bradycardia and respiratory failure and therefore above measures should be observed.
- *Imaging*: CT scan of the thorax to demonstrate thymoma or thymic hyperplasia.

MANAGEMENT
- Medical:
  - o *Symptomatic*: Cholinesterase inhibitors (pyridostigmine) increase the amount of Ach at the NMJ by diminishing Ach metabolism and thereby increasing Ach exposure to the remaining receptors available. Side effects are due to muscarinic stimulation (nausea, vomiting, diarrhoea, abdominal cramps and increased salivation). In addition, overtreatment can lead to increased weakness. Differentiation from myasthenic crisis related to under-treatment versus overtreatment can be made using an edrophonium test.
  - o *Immune therapy*: Corticosteroids can be used in cases of generalised and ocular MG. Steroids, however, can produce an initial worsening in the clinical condition and should therefore be started at a low dose with gradual increase and close monitoring of the patient. Other immunosuppressants such as azathioprine are employed to spare long-term steroids. Intravenous immunoglobulin or plasmapheresis may be utilised in cases of severe exacerbation of MG.
- *Surgical*: Thymectomy is carried out in young patients (<50 years old) to improve the chance of remission. Thymic tumours such as thymoma warrant thymectomy.

> *Remember: Corticosteroids can produce an initial worsening in the clinical condition, so start at a low dose and increase gradually.*

COMPLICATIONS
- Myasthenic crisis with severe weakness producing bulbar and respiratory failure.
- The above can be characterised by both the increased risk of aspiration pneumonia and the decreasing forced vital capacity (FVC) with a figure of less than 1.5 L prompting need for possible ventilation.
- *Treatment*: Supportive with serial monitoring of FVC and movement of patients to a high dependency/ITU setting.

PROGNOSIS

- Most patients have near normal lifespan, spontaneous remission can occur.
- Thymectomy in younger patients can lead to remission in 25% of cases and clinical improvement in a further 50%.

DIFFERENTIAL DIAGNOSES (TABLE 27.1)

Table 27.1 Differential diagnoses with points to note for MG

Clinical conditions	Points to note
Lambert–Eaton myasthenic syndrome (LEMS)	Occurs as an autoimmune disorder or paraneoplastic syndrome in association with carcinoma of lung (small cell), prostate and breast
	Antibodies directed against voltage-gated *presynaptic* calcium channels preventing release of Ach (compare with MG)
	Autonomic involvement (dry mouth and constipation) and subacute weakness (proximal muscles of pelvic and shoulder girdles) with gait difficulty
	Rare involvement of ocular muscles
	Clinically hyporeflexia with increased strength and reflexes postexertion (reflex potentiation)
	cMAP *increment* (as opposed to *decrement* in MG) on repetitive stimulation
	Treatment: 3,4-diaminopyridine and i.v. immunoglobulin
	Close follow-up required as syndrome may precede the onset of the malignancy by years
	Careful search for occult malignancy, consider whole-body FDG–PET scan
Medications, for example aminoglycosides, beta-blockers, calcium channel blockers, steroids, D-penicillamine and lithium	Take adequate drug history. All these drugs can affect the NMJ
Botulism (*Clostridium botulinum*)	Due to botulinum toxin binding to voltage-gated calcium channel of presynaptic membrane leading to fatal paralysis
	Related to wound infection with the bacterium (seen in intravenous drug users) or consumption of toxin in inadequately preserved foods
Polymyositis (Chapter 28)	An inflammatory muscle disease with subacute or chronic onset in adults (50–70 years) affecting proximal muscles in limbs; oesophageal, trunk, neck and pharyngeal muscles with associated muscle tenderness
	Diagnosis relies on markedly elevated creatine kinase, EMG and muscle biopsy
	There may be an associated underlying malignancy especially in cases of dermatomyositis in older patients (>40 years)

28   Diseases of the muscle

INTRODUCTION   Muscle diseases produce skeletal muscle weakness and frequently lead to cardiorespiratory complications. Their age of onset is extremely wide; patients may die young or there may be lifelong motor and cardiorespiratory disability or late onset of muscle weakness.

Muscle diseases typically present with wasting, weakness, sometimes pain and potential pseudo-hypertrophy or abnormal muscle contraction. They can be classified by considering when and where the problem originates.

Muscle diseases can be considered to be acquired or congenital. Acquired causes include inflammatory myopathies (Table 28.1) and drug- or toxin-induced myopathy as with statins or alcohol. Congenital causes include muscular dystrophies (a collection of inherited progressive disorders characterized by muscle destruction and eventual replacement by fibrous tissue and fat, for example Duchenne, Becker's and myotonic muscular dystrophy) (Table 28.2); skeletal muscle channelopathies (disorders of muscle membrane excitability linked to mutations in various ion channel genes, for example hypokalaemic periodic paralysis); metabolic myopathies, including mitochondrial disorders (confined to muscle or form part of a multi-system disorder), disorders of fatty acid metabolism (disorders of B oxidation leading to inadequate energy supply to muscle and accumulation of toxic intermediates and carnitine and co-enzyme A depletion) and disorders of carbohydrate metabolism (malfunction in muscle glycogen metabolism, for example as seen in acid maltase deficiency or McArdle's disease); and finally congenital myopathy (uncommon, for example Nemaline myopathy).

APPROACH TO DIAGNOSIS   Distinguishing myopathies from peripheral neuropathies, anterior horn cell diseases (e.g. motor neurone disease) and neuromuscular junction disorders (e.g. myasthenic syndromes) requires careful clinical evaluation supplemented by investigations including neurophysiological testing, imaging, muscle biopsy and genetic exploration.

Determining aetiology of a myopathy depends upon a careful history and examination to elicit distinguishing features, including family history, age of onset and the rate of progression (including eliciting if symptoms are persistent or episodic), and the presence of additional features such as muscle aching and pain (myalgia) or urine turning black (myoglobinuria). Any provoking or relieving factors should be noted. From examination, the pattern of muscle involvement (facial, bulbar and, if involving limbs, whether proximal or distal and symmetric or asymmetric) will give further clues as will additional examination findings such as wasting, pseudo-hypertrophy, delayed relaxation after voluntary contraction (myotonia) and involuntary, spontaneous quivering of muscle bundles (myokymia).

Many of the above-mentioned muscle diseases are outside the scope of this book. The important acquired muscle diseases, however, include the inflammatory myopathies which are treatable and are covered in more detail in the following section. Remember neurologists are often asked to assess patients with weakness, where this is found to be secondary to ageing, immobility, critical illness or cancer.

The treatable inflammatory Mmyopathies

DEFINITION   Polymyositis is a progressive inflammatory striated muscle disease in adults involving proximal muscles symmetrically in limbs, trunk, pharyngeal and oesophageal muscles.

Dermatomyositis is characterised by symptoms of polymyositis as well as cutaneous involvement.

Remember: Symmetric involvement of proximal limb muscles is an important feature of both conditions.

EPIDEMIOLOGY   Usually affects patients between 50 and 70 years of age; M:F = 1:2. Dermatomyositis can also affect children (5–14 years old).

AETIOLOGY
- Idiopathic inflammatory myopathy (possibly autoimmune).

ASSOCIATIONS/RISK FACTORS
- Occurs as an isolated syndrome or as part of a collagen vascular disease (polyarteritis nodosa), sarcoidosis.
- Increased risk of malignancy in both, particularly in dermatomyositis (ovarian and lymphoma).

Remember: The association between malignancy and polymyositis and especially dermatomyositis.

PATHOLOGY/PATHOGENESIS
- In both conditions, immune-mediated muscle inflammation and damage to blood vessels occur; in dermatomyositis, dermal microvasculature is also affected.

HISTORY   Inflammatory myopathies usually have a subacute or chronic (weeks to months) onset with patients complaining of proximal limb weakness (difficulty in climbing stairs or arising from a chair or raising arms). With advanced disease, patients may also complain of difficulties in breathing and swallowing (dysphagia). In addition, painful joints may be reported and characteristic rash may be seen in dermatomyositis, as described below.

EXAMINATION
- Proximal limb weakness with muscle tenderness, normal sensory examination and reflexes.
- *Dermatomyositis:* Heliotrope rash (periorbital purple rash), shawl sign (macular rash over shoulders, upper chest and back), Gottron's papules (a papular scaly rash over knuckles, elbows and knees) and erythema in nail-fold due to dilated capillary loops.
- *Others (with both conditions):* Fever; myocarditis and cardiac conduction defects (arrhythmias); evidence of interstitial lung disease and aspiration pneumonia.

Remember: Despite the similarities between polymyositis and dermatomyositis, they are distinct clinical entities.

INVESTIGATIONS
- *Blood tests:* Increased muscle enzymes (CK blood level often in the thousands) and elevated inflammatory markers (CRP, ESR) and plasma viscosity. Association with anti-Mi-2 and anti-Jo1 autoantibodies.
- *EMG:* Demonstrates fibrillation potentials; ECG: arrhythmias or conduction defects.
- *Muscle biopsy (diagnostic):* Inflammatory changes and fibres in different stages of necrosis and regeneration.

MANAGEMENT

- *Steroids:* High-dose corticosteroids (prednisolone) decreased after 4–6 weeks to a lower maintenance dose. Serial CK and inflammatory marker measurements in combination with continuing clinical assessment allows monitoring of disease activity and tailoring of treatment.
- *Other immunosuppressants:* Such as azathioprine or methotrexate can be used over the long term, particularly in resistant cases.

COMPLICATIONS

- Respiratory (pneumonia) and swallowing difficulties (aspiration pneumonia) related to advanced disease.
- *Malignancy:* Patients should have an annual examination and undergo investigations like US of pelvis and abdomen, CXR, breast mammogram and flexible sigmoidoscopy (plus or minus CT of the chest, abdomen and pelvis with or without a whole-body ^{18}FDG–PET scan) as appropriate based on age and sex; this is due to increased risk of developing malignancy (breast, lung or ovarian).
- Steroid-related myopathy and side effects.

PROGNOSIS

- Twenty per cent 5-year mortality rate, predominantly related to associated malignancy or pulmonary complications.

DIFFERENTIAL DIAGNOSES

Table 28.1 Other conditions of note producing an acquired myopathy

Clinical conditions	Points to note
Systemic metabolic/endocrine disturbance, for example Cushing's disease, thyroid abnormalities, electrolyte disturbance (low calcium, magnesium and potassium), renal and liver failure	Can be associated with proximal muscle weakness. Appropriate blood tests according to suspicion of underlying cause. EMG, CK and biopsy results should be normal
Drugs including steroids, statins and alcohol	Complete drug history. Symptoms usually resolve with discontinuation of offending cause
Infections, for example HIV, and connective tissue disorders	Pertinent past medical history and associated clinical features. Microbiological and immunological blood tests
Inclusion body myositis	The most common acquired muscle disease in >50 years old, three times more frequent in men than women. Due to cytotoxic T-cell-mediated attack. Early involvement of deep finger flexors, foot extensors and quadriceps is an important clue to the diagnosis. Relentlessly progressive and typically unresponsive to immunosuppressants

Remember: An episode of acute myopathy with marked muscle damage may result in myoglobinaemia and myoglobinuria (leading to acute renal tubular necrosis) and may be secondary to burns, viral infections (e.g. HIV), drugs like statins and trauma.

Table 28.2 Common inherited muscular dystrophies

Clinical conditions	Points to note
Muscular dystrophy	Inherited conditions (X-linked recessive)
Duchenne muscular dystrophy	Related to deficiency of dystrophin, a cytoskeletal protein
	Onset in males at 3–5 years
	Mainly affects axial and proximal muscles (difficulty in walking with waddling gait, Gower's manoeuvre[a] and pseudo-hypertrophy of gastrocnemius)
	Low IQ in up to 30%
	Negative dystrophin immunostain and fibre degeneration on muscle biopsy; elevated CK and polyphasic potentials on EMG
	Survival into mid-20s (death from respiratory complications)
	Physiotherapy to prevent contractures and respiratory infections
Becker muscular dystrophy	Onset at 5–15 years
	Dystrophin present, but abnormal
	Milder course with calf pseudo-hypertrophy; mental retardation is uncommon
	Elevated CK
	Survival into 30–40s
Myotonic dystrophy	Autosomal dominant disorder
	Caused by a trinucleotide repeat sequence on chromosome 19
	A multi-system disorder with frontal balding, bilateral ptosis, myopathic facies, muscle thinning and wasting, cataracts, testicular atrophy and mild mental retardation
	Myotonia is observed following voluntary contraction, for example clenching the fist followed by attempted rapid opening
	Percussion myotonia and tongue myotonia may also be seen
	ECG abnormalities are found in the majority and patients can suffer sudden cardiac death. Associated problems include diabetes which should be looked for. General anaesthetics should be administered with care

[a]Gower's manoeuvre refers to the act of use of hands to push off the thighs while rising from the floor.

29   Alzheimer's disease and other dementia syndromes

DEFINITION   Dementia is a clinical term describing progressive impairment of multiple cognitive domains such as memory, judgement and naming. This is associated with a deterioration in day-to-day functioning, but without impaired consciousness. Alzheimer's disease (AD) is the commonest cause; other primary causes include frontotemporal lobar degeneration leading to frontotemporal dementia (FTD), Lewy Body dementia (LBD) and Prion disease.

EPIDEMIOLOGY
- Dementia affects as many as 10% of the population over 65 years, with over half of those (~60%) due to AD.
- LBD accounts for 15–20% of all dementia cases with the remainder due to vascular dementia (VaD), FTD, CJD and others.

AETIOLOGY
- *Genetic:* Genetic factors play a role in both familial and sporadic cases of AD. Familial AD has a prevalence of less than 0.1%, has a younger age of onset (<65 years) and an autosomal dominant inheritance. Point mutations in three genes associated with amyloid processing, the amyloid precursor protein (APP) (on chromosome 21), presenilin 1 (PS1) (on chromosome 14) and presenilin 2 (PS2) (on chromosome 1) are known to be causative.
- *Apolipoprotein E (ApoE):* This gene is thought to be important in the earlier development of sporadic (non-familial) AD; there are three allelic variants, including E2–E4. Possession of two E4 alleles is thought to increase the risk of developing AD.

ASSOCIATIONS/RISK FACTORS
- *Increasing age*: Approximately 10% of people over 75 years of age will develop dementia rising to 20% over age 85 years; rare under the age of 60 years.
- Family history of dementia in first-degree relative (see above).
- *Level of educational achievement*: Lower levels of achievement and occupational attainment have been associated with an increased risk of developing AD.

PATHOLOGY/PATHOGENESIS
- Cerebral atrophy tends to involve the hippocampus and medial temporal lobe structures first, before affecting the rest of the cortex.
- *Neuropathological examination*: Intracellular neurofibrillary tangles and extracellular amyloid plaques. These pathological processes result in biological changes in the brain, including neurotransmitter loss, dendritic pruning of neurons and cell death. This forms the basis of use of acetylcholinesterase inhibitors for symptomatic improvement in AD.

Remember: Neurofibrillary tangles and amyloid plaques are features on neuropathological examination in AD.

HISTORY
- In AD, symptoms of memory loss are the commonest initial complaint. Forgetfulness is often reported by family or friends and work performance may decline. If memory loss is the only deficit and day-to-day functioning is preserved, a patient is given the diagnosis of mild cognitive impairment (MCI); 80% of these patients will develop AD over a 5 year period.
- If an individual has memory loss and further cognitive decline, for example speech disturbance, or impaired judgement, affecting their day-to-day functioning, they may be

given a diagnosis of AD (according to certain criteria). Characteristically, personality is preserved until later in the disease process which can help differentiate AD from other types of dementia (e.g. FTD).

- As the disease progresses over a 6–8 year period, patients display severe global intellectual decline and loss of ability to care for themselves, including incontinence.

Remember: The history of onset and progression is important in dementia syndromes as a gradual onset with steady progression points towards a degenerative condition as opposed to a sudden onset and stepwise deterioration suggesting VaD or cognitive decline of cerebrovascular aetiology. Collateral history from friends or family is very important in making a diagnosis.

EXAMINATION *delirium*

- Conscious level is not impaired. MMSE is essential (scores usually less than 24/30) and demonstrates deficits in two or more areas of cognition (e.g. memory and naming).
- In the earlier stages of AD, a neurological examination is usually normal; in later stages of the disease, primitive reflexes, for example pout, palmomental, and grasp may emerge with increased tone (gegenhalten pattern). The presence of major neurological deficits suggests other possible diagnoses for dementia (see Section 'Differential Diagnoses').

INVESTIGATIONS

- No definitive diagnostic test; neuropathological examination at autopsy provides the definitive diagnosis.
- An important role of investigations, in addition to clinical examination, is to exclude structural or reversible and treatable causes for dementia.
- *Blood tests*: FBC; biochemical profile including calcium, renal and liver function; B12 and folate levels; thyroid function tests; thyroid autoantibodies; syphilis serology; inflammatory markers like ESR and CRP; serum electrophoresis and autoimmune screen. HIV serology could be requested if clinically indicated.
- EEG can exclude symptoms of memory loss due to temporal lobe epilepsy, and can identify the loss of alpha rhythm, a characteristic of AD.
- Imaging should include a chest X-ray and neuroimaging, with MRI the investigation of choice. This will demonstrate cerebral atrophy particularly affecting medial temporal lobe structures (hippocampus and parahippocampal gyrus). Other features include enlarged ventricles in proportion to cerebral atrophy and prominent cerebral sulci.
- LP is not a routine investigation, but should be carried out in individuals presenting at a young age or where another aetiology, for example prion disease, is suspected. S100 and 14.3.3 proteins, when present in CSF, can support a diagnosis of CJD, in combination with other features. LP should only be performed after imaging studies have excluded an intracranial space-occupying lesion due to the risk of cerebral herniation.
- Neuropsychological evaluation at intervals assesses disease progression, as well as provides a useful baseline for cognitive functioning.

Remember: LP if indicated should only be performed after imaging studies have excluded an intracranial space occupying lesion due to risk of herniation.

MANAGEMENT

- Treatment of AD is largely supportive. Provision of social support and help for the carers and the patient with the resulting economic burden is one of the major challenges facing the NHS in the United Kingdom.

- There are several cholinesterase inhibitors (e.g. Donepezil) licensed for treatment in mild and moderate dementia in AD to improve cognitive function. These do not affect the underlying disease process.
- Atypical neuroleptics (e.g. quetiapine) in lowest effective dose can be used to treat agitation or psychotic symptoms. Antidepressants in a proportion of patients are useful in treating any coexistent depression.

> *Remember: Patients with LBD can be exquisitely sensitive to neuroleptic administration and develop severe akinesia.*

COMPLICATIONS
- Susceptible to acute confusional states which may be triggered by trauma; infection of the urinary tract or chest among others or due to polypharmacy and the resultant interactions between medications. Careful clinical evaluation should be carried out prior to treating.

PROGNOSIS
- The mean life expectancy after diagnosis is approximately 7 years. Less than 3% of patients will survive more than 14 years.

DIFFERENTIAL DIAGNOSES (TABLE 29.1)

Table 29.1 Differential diagnoses with points to note for dementia syndromes

Clinical conditions	Points to note
Lewy Body dementia	Characterised by cortical Lewy Bodies, also present in substantia nigra
	Prominent features include fluctuations in cognitive status, visual hallucinations and sensitivity to neuroleptics, particularly typical antipsychotics which can cause severe akinetic state
	Extrapyramidal features may be present
	Rivastigmine (anticholinesterase) may be tried to improve cognition
Vascular dementia	Occurs as a result of multiple small strokes or vascular insults
	Sudden onset and stepwise deterioration are characteristic with possible presence of focal CNS signs such as hemiparesis or visual field loss (compare with AD where these do not occur)
	Associated with vascular risk factors, for example hypertension or history of strokes
Frontotemporal dementia	Causes 5–10% of dementia
	Characteristic neuronal inclusions called Pick Bodies in a third of cases
	Selective atrophy of frontal and temporal lobes
	Features include overactivity and disinhibition progressing to apathy and withdrawal as disease progresses
	Occasionally can coexist with MND

Intracranial neoplasm and other structural lesions (Chapters 33 and 36)	Cognitive impairment may occur over a period of months related to generalised mass effect or hydrocephalus from a neoplasm
	Lesions can include meningiomas or chronic subdural haematomas associated with falls, use of antiplatelet drugs and fluctuating cognition in the elderly
Infective causes	CJD: Prion disease associated with rapidly progressive dementia, myoclonus and diagnostic periodic sharp wave on EEG. Usually leads to death within 12 months
	HIV dementia: Commonest form of dementia in young population. HIV serology in suspected patients
	Other causes: Syphilis, Whipple's disease, *Cryptococcus*, progressive multifocal leucoencephalopathy (PML) associated with JC virus
Toxic and metabolic causes	Chronic alcohol abuse
	Vitamin deficiency: Niacin deficiency leads to pellagra, a syndrome of cognitive impairment and extrapyramidal rigidity. Others implicated include thiamine deficiency causing Wernicke's encephalopathy[a] and Korsakoff's psychosis; B12 deficiency
Normal pressure hydrocephalus (NPH) (Chapter 37)	Hydrocephalus can cause cognitive decline irrespective of aetiology. NPH, a type of communicating hydrocephalus in >60 years old, results in the triad of (not pathognomonic) gait disturbance, dementia (memory impairment and bradyphrenia) and urinary incontinence
	CT and MRI may help in diagnosis
	Evaluation of gait and cognition after a period of external lumbar CSF drainage may also facilitate diagnosis
	Symptoms often reversible with a CSF shunt, so it is important not to miss diagnosis
	May coexist with other dementias particularly AD and VaD

[a]Wernicke's encephalopathy related to thiamine deficiency: The classical triad (not present in all cases) includes gait ataxia, opthalmoplegia (lateral rectus palsy and nystagmus) and encephalopathy characterised by global confusion. Korsakoff's syndrome or psychosis, characterised by amnesia (retrograde and anterograde) may follow encephalopathy.

Alcoholics are susceptible owing to malnourishment among other factors. Treatment: In suspected cases, administer thiamine intravenously. Give thiamine before glucose administration in patients with thiamine deficiency as intravenous glucose can precipitate Wernicke's encephalopathy.

30 Raised intracranial pressure and herniation syndromes

DEFINITION   Intracranial pressure (ICP) is the pressure within the intracranial compartment. It is distributed evenly throughout the intracranial cavity and corresponds to the pressure in the brain tissue and CSF. It is measured relative to the foramen of Monro (usually approximated to the external auditory meatus). In normal supine adults the ICP is 5–15 mmHg (often negative readings in the upright position). Readings can transiently be much higher during coughing, straining or valsalva (over 50 mmHg). In infants ICP is <5 mmHg. The lumbar CSF pressure in a supine patient equates to the ICP.

- Raised ICP will result in brain damage only if cerebral blood flow (CBF) is compromised.
- CBF = Cerebral perfusion pressure (CPP)/cerebral vascular resistance (CVR).
- The CVR is controlled by cerebral autoregulation (changes in vessel calibre in response to changes in either systemic blood pressure (constricting when high) or metabolic changes (e.g. CO_2 increase causes vasodilatation)).
- CPP = Mean arterial pressure (MAP) − ICP. The CPP is normally >50 mmHg.
- If CPP is severely reduced it will result in impaired CBF leading to cerebral ischaemic damage (occurs when CBF is <20 mL/100 g of brain tissue/min).

AETIOLOGY OF RAISED ICP

Intracranial mass lesion:
- *Tumour*: (see Chapter 36).
- *Infection*: Abscess/subdural empyema (pus in subdural space)/tuberculoma/hydatid cyst (see Chapter 22).
- *Haematoma*: Traumatic or spontaneous (see Chapters 33 and 34).

Increase in CSF volume:
- Obstructive or communicating hydrocephalus (see Chapter 37).

Increase in cerebral blood volume:
- Venous outflow obstruction (e.g. cerebral venous sinus thrombosis).
- Vasodilatation (e.g. reactive hyperaemia due to loss of autoregulation following head injury).

Cerebral oedema:
- An increase in the volume of the brain due to an accumulation of 'brain water' either in or around cells (neurons and glia).
- Affected brain is more hypodense (darker) on CT.
- Two main types—vasogenic and cytotoxic.
- Both are often present in variable proportions particularly in trauma and following ischaemic insults.
- *Vasogenic oedema*:
  - Secondary to breakdown of blood-brain barrier, leakage of (normally excluded) intravascular proteins and fluid into the cerebral interstitial space.
  - Primarily affects *white matter*.
  - Seen around tumours, abscesses.
  - Can occur in late stages of cerebral ischaemia due to ischaemic damage to cerebral vessels.
  - Posterior reversible encephalopathy syndrome (PRES) is a type of vasogenic oedema which often arises secondary to malignant hypertension.
  - Altitude sickness (high altitude cerebral oedema (HACE)).
  - Seen on MRI as elevated apparent diffusion coefficient (ADC) (i.e. increased water diffusion).
  - *Responds to dexamethasone therapy.*

- *Cytotoxic oedema*:
  - ○ Increase in intracellular fluid in glia (particularly astrocytes) and neurons due to failure of cellular metabolism (ATP-dependent ion channels). Predominantly affects *grey matter*.
  - ○ Commonest cause is early cerebral ischaemia (failure of oxygen delivery to brain tissue), for example stroke; near drowning; cardiac arrest; carbon monoxide poisoning.
  - ○ Drugs and toxins, for example hepatic encephalopathy (secondary to elevated ammonia); isoniazid.
  - ○ Seen on MRI as reduced ADC (decreased water diffusion).
  - ○ *Not helped by dexamethasone*.
- *Interstitial oedema*:
  - ○ Secondary to obstructive hydrocephalus which causes transependymal bulk flow of CSF from ventricle into adjacent white matter.
  - ○ Oedema predominantly affects periventricular white matter.

Remember: Vasogenic and not cytotoxic oedema is helped by dexamethasone therapy.

Prevention of normal skull growth (children):
  - ○ Multisutural synostosis (premature fusion of skull sutures), for example Crouzon's syndrome.

PATHOLOGY/PATHOGENESIS
Monro–Kellie doctrine:

Remember: The cranial compartment (the skull) is of a fixed volume. Any increase in volume of one of the intracranial contents (blood (intravascular or haematoma), CSF or brain tissue (oedema/tumour/abscess)) must be compensated by a decrease in another.

- In normal circumstances, small increases in volume of contents are initially accommodated by the following:
  - ○ A reduction in ventricular CSF-by (i) shifting it from the ventricles to the expandable spinal theca and (ii) increasing its absorption (which is pressure dependent).
  - ○ A decrease in cerebral blood volume (predominantly venous).
- In the longer term further compensation can occur due to a reduction in extracelluar fluid volume causing a further (reversible) decrease in brain parenchymal volume.
- When the above compensatory mechanisms are exceeded the ICP will rise.

Remember: Infants are the exception as their skull sutures have not fused. In response to an increase in volume their sutures separate (diastasis) and the cranial vault enlarges to accommodate the increase in volume. bulging fontanelles.

HISTORY
- *Headache*: Global headache; usually persistent, may be relieved on standing or by vomiting; may wake from sleep in early morning due to headache; worse on coughing or straining.

Remember: This may be the only symptom/sign in mildly elevated ICP.

- *Vomiting.*
- *Drowsiness.*
- *Confusion.*

EXAMINATION

- *Depressed level of consciousness*: Assessed using Glasgow Coma Score (see Appendix 2). Correlates with severity of raised ICP.
- *Eye signs*: Papilloedema is not always present but if found is a reliable indicator of elevated ICP; may damage vision in more severe and/or prolonged cases resulting in optic atrophy causing enlarged blind spot, constricted visual fields, decreased visual acuity. Bilateral (usually) CN VI (abducens) nerve palsies (*false localising sign*, long intracranial course of VI nerve makes it susceptible to stretch with raised ICP).
- Foster Kennedy Syndrome: mass lesion (usually an olfactory groove meningioma) compressing one optic nerve – causing atrophy, with papilloedema on contralateral side due to raised ICP from tumour.
- *Cushing's triad*: Hypertension, bradycardia and respiratory irregularity. Only seen with severely elevated ICP usually in comatose patients.
- *Infants*: Full or tense fontanelle; enlarged head (plot on growth chart); dilated scalp veins.

> *Remember: the significance of CN VI palsy as a false localising sign in the setting of raised ICP.*

INVESTIGATIONS

- Symptoms OR signs of raised ICP should prompt neuroimaging (*CT or MRI brain*). In significant head trauma (see Chapters 32, 33, 34), or in cases associated with a depressed level of consciousness an immediate CT should be the first investigation performed; contrast may be required to identify a mass lesion. In non-traumatic cases without depressed consciousness an urgent MRI scan may provide additional diagnostic information.
- In non-traumatic cases, *if no mass lesion is identified on imaging and the cerebral aqueduct is patent on imaging* a lumbar puncture can be performed to measure the CSF pressure and obtain CSF for analysis.
- ICP monitoring can be performed in a neurosurgical unit either via a ventricular catheter (allowing therapeutic CSF drainage if required) or an implanted parenchymal transducer.

MANAGEMENT

> *Remember: In patients with raised ICP the principles are to (i) reduce ICP and (ii) protect the brain from damage due to impaired cerebral blood flow.*

Reducing ICP: The principles of ICP reduction are based around the Morno–Kellie Doctrine, you can do either of the following:

Reduce the volume of the intracranial contents:

- Surgical excision/drainage of any mass lesion (tumour, haematoma, abscess etc).
- Surgical drainage of CSF from the ventricle (even if hydrocephalus is not present this may still help reduce ICP).
- Optimise venous drainage of the brain:
  - Elevate head of bed to 30 degrees
  - If cause of raised ICP is cerebral venous sinus thrombosis consider thrombolysis.
- Prevent hyperaemic vasodilatation: maintain pCO_2 at 4.0–4.5 kPa.

- 'Shrink' the brain:
  - *Osmotic agents* (*reduce brain interstitial fluid*): i.v. bolus of 20% mannitol or hypertonic saline.
  - *Steroids* (*dexamethasone*): Reduce vasogenic oedema around tumours and cerebral abscesses (not helpful in trauma or ischaemic injury).
  - Brief (minutes) hyperventilation (to pCO_2 3.5–4.0 kPa) can transiently reduce cerebral blood volume to offset 'spikes' of raised ICP in ventilated patients.

Increase the volume of the intracranial compartment:

- Surgical decompressive craniectomy: Removing the skull vault and surgically expanding the dural sac to allow the brain to swell without raising the ICP.
- *Brain resection*: In trauma, a non-dominant partial temporal or frontal lobectomy can be considered, particularly if those areas are badly contused.

Cerebral protection:

- *Intubation and ventilation*: Ensures adequate cerebral oxygenation and control of CO_2. Certain anaesthetic agents such as propofol also have neuroprotective qualities.
- *Reduce brain metabolism*:
  - High does barbiturate therapy (thiopentone coma) can be used for intractable raised ICP; it is given until 'burst suppression' seen on EEG (i.e. 'shuts down' neuronal activity) reducing the cerebral oxygen requirements of the brain tissue.
  - *Cerebral cooling*: moderate hypothermia reduces brain oxygen requirements.

COMPLICATIONS

Visual loss: Severe and prolonged papilloedema can result in visual loss due to optic atrophy.

Cerebral herniation:

Type	Causes	Clinical findings	Progression
Subfalcine (syn. 'midline shift')	Unilateral supratentorial mass lesion causes herniation across midline below falx cerebri	Often asymptomatic. Can result in contralateral hydrocephalus of lateral ventricle, further exacerbating raised ICP. If severe can cause kinking and infarction of distal ipsilateral anterior cerebral artery causing contralateral leg weakness	Can progress to uncal herniation
Uncal (lateral tentorial)	Unilateral, supratentorial mass lesion causes the medial edge of the temporal lobe (known as the uncus) to herniate through the tentorial hiatus.	Compression of IIIrd nerve causes ipsilateral pupillary dilatation that is unreactive to light (a 'fixed' pupil). Kinking of the posterior cerebral artery can cause a homonymous haemianopia. Pressure from the contralateral edge of the tentorium against the cerebral peduncle (resulting in an indentation of the peduncle known as 'Kernohan's notch') can cause an ipsilateral hemiparesis (a 'false localising sign'). Pressure on the midbrain reticular formation results in deterioration in the level of consciousness	Can progress to central and then tonsillar herniation
Central tentorial (transtentorial)	Diffuse bilateral hemisphere swelling, hydrocephalus or midline mass lesions	Distortion and ischaemia of diencephalic and midbrain structures causes coma. Pupils may initially be small later becoming fixed and mid-sized. Distortion	Can lead to tonsillar herniation

CN3 – Parasym
fixed
dilated
(a nopposed symp)

	cause vertical displacement of the diencephalon through the tentorial hiatus.	of the pituitary stalk may cause diabetes insipidus. Pressure on the upper midbrain (tectum) can result in a loss of up-gaze (Parinaud's syndrome). Bilateral kinking of the posterior cerebral arteries can result in bilateral occipital lobe infarction and cortical blindness. 'Duret' haemorrhages in the ventral midbrain seen on imaging	
Upward cerebellar	Posterior fossa mass lesion causes upward herniation of the rostral cerebellum through tentorial hiatus	Can result in kinking and ischaemia of the superior cerebellar arteries causing cerebellar infarction or venous obstruction of the vein of Galen causing haemorrhagic venous infarction of the diencephalon. Clinical effects variable but include coma (diencephalic or midbrain damage); small, minimally reactive pupils ('pontine' pupils). Obstructive hydrocephalus from cerebral aqueduct compression.	Usually associated with or leads to tonsillar herniation
Tonsillar	Can arise as a result of progression of herniation from a supratentorial lesion or can arise directly from an expanding posterior fossa mass.	Severe depression of consciousness, Cushing's triad (see above) and eventually cardio-respiratory arrest. Chronic tonsillar herniation ('acquired Chiari I malformation') can cause neck stiffness, head tilt, lower cranial nerve neuropathies, hydrocephalus (due to fourth ventricular CSF outflow obstruction) and syringomyelia (due to obstruction of CSF flow through the foramen magnum)	Usually rapidly fatal in the acute setting

PROGNOSIS   Dependent on the underlying cause of raised ICP and whether the elevated ICP has resulted in any cerebral ischaemic damage to the brain.

Notes on differential diagnoses (see also Chapter 31 on coma)
Intracranial Hypotension: Also causes headaches worse on coughing and straining and can be associated with vomiting and diplopia, however headaches are relieved on lying flat and worse on standing.
Pseudopapilloedema: Occurs due to small 'crowded' hyperopic disc or optic disc drusen.
Papillitis: Infective or inflammatory conditions such as optic neuritis, sarcoidosis and syphilis causing 'true' disc oedema due to a direct effect on the optic nerve, but without associated raised ICP.

31 Coma and brainstem death

DEFINITION   GCS ≤ 8 is a generally accepted definition of coma. Patients are therefore unconscious and unable to obey commands.

AETIOLOGY   Causes can be considered under diffuse and focal category.
* *Diffuse:*
    o *Toxic*: Alcohol abuse and overdose with drugs, for example opiates.
    o *Metabolic/endocrine*: Hypoglycaemia, hyperosmolar non-ketotic coma and diabetic ketoacidosis in diabetes; electrolyte disturbances, including hyponatraemia or hypernatraemia and hypercalcaemia; renal failure leading to uraemia; hepatic failure causing encephalopathy and raised ammonia; and myxoedema coma.
    o *Vascular*: SAH, hypertensive encephalopathy and vasculitis.
    o *Ischaemia*: Anoxic encephalopathy (post-CPR) and carbon monoxide poisoning.
    o *Infection*: Meningitis, encephalitis and generalised sepsis.
    o Posttraumatic following severe head injury.
    o *Epilepsy*: Postictal state and status epilepticus.
    o *Others*: Carbon dioxide narcosis and Wernicke's encephalopathy.
* *Focal (can be supratentorial or infratentorial):*
    o Infarction.
    o *Neoplasm*: Primary or secondary.
    o *Infection*: Intraparenchymal abscess, subdural empyema and herpes simplex encephalitis.
    o Haematoma (subdural or extradural) and traumatic contusions.

ASSOCIATIONS/RISK FACTORS   See under aetiology.

PATHOLOGY/PATHOGENESIS   Maintenance of consciousness relies upon an intact reticular activating system (RAS). Fibres for RAS start in the pons and ascend through mid-brain to terminate in thalamus and hypothalamus. An infratentorial lesion may directly affect the RAS while a supratentorial lesion may cause cortical dysfunction and transtentorial herniation leading to brainstem distortion and coma. Diffuse or metabolic causes result in coma by impairing cerebral metabolism.

HISTORY   It is important to obtain any relevant history from witnesses, ambulance staff, police, relatives or friends.

EXAMINATION   A sequential examination can proceed as follows:
* Airway (risk of compromised airway, therefore check need for airways adjunct or formal intubation and ventilation: inform on-call anaesthetist).
* Breathing (respiratory rate, rhythm and character, for example Cheyne–Stokes, hyperventilation, apneustic or ataxic pattern due to progressive herniation).
* Circulation (pulse rate, BP, rhythm—check for evidence of Cushing's triad ($\uparrow$BP, $\downarrow$PR and irregular respiratory pattern).
* GCS (see Appendix 2).
* Temperature and glucose (fingerstick).
* *Appearance and inspection on exposure*: Meningococcal purpuric rash, alcoholic fetor, jaundice, otorrhoea or blood from ear.
* *Eyes*: Pupils (size, symmetry and reaction), extraocular movements (spontaneous; internuclear opthalmoplegia; vestibulo-ocular reflex or caloric test; oculocephalic reflex or doll's head manoeuvre) and fundoscopy (papilloedema).
* *Brainstem function*: Corneal reflex and gag reflex.
* *Motor*: Check tone, reflexes and plantar response and note any asymmetry. Response to pain as decorticate posturing (implying lesion at cortical or subcortical level) or decerebrate posturing (brainstem pathology) should be noted.
* Full general examination.

Remember: Pupillary examination is invaluable in comatose patients with the presence of equal and reactive pupils usually indicating a diffuse or toxic/metabolic cause. Note however that atropine and glutethimide can result in fixed/dilated pupils, while opiates lead to small pupils with sluggish reaction to light. A unilateral fixed and dilated pupil usually suggests oculomotor nerve palsy due to progressive herniation from a focal, supratentorial mass lesion.

INVESTIGATIONS   These should be tailored according to the results of examination and evaluation of the patient indicating either a focal or a diffuse lesion for coma.
- *Imaging:* CT head is imperative if a focal lesion is suspected or if there is any history of trauma.
- *Blood tests:* FBC, U & E (especially sodium), serum osmolality, LFT, glucose, calcium, blood alcohol and ammonia levels, ABG, blood culture, toxicology screen or drug levels including antiepileptic drug (AED) levels if indicated.
- *Lumbar puncture (LP):* Useful for excluding meningitis or encephalitis when suspected in the presence of meningeal signs or fever.
- *EEG:* May demonstrate non-convulsive status or generalised changes suggesting meningoencephalitis or a metabolic abnormality.
- *Urine:* Routine MC & S, toxicology screen and osmolality.

Remember: LP should not be performed prior to imaging of the head if a focal lesion is suspected due to risk of herniation.

MANAGEMENT   In comatose patients, initial management is instituted parallel to assessment and evaluation and again tailored towards the suspected underlying cause.
- Stabilisation of **a**irway, **b**reathing and **c**irculation with regular monitoring of respiratory and cardiovascular parameters and pupillary size.
- Administration of glucose intravenously (unless definitely known to be normal) and thiamine (Wernicke's encephalopathy).
- Administer naloxone (opiate overdose) or flumazenil (benzodiazepine overdose).
- Initiate measures to lower ICP (e.g. head up, pCO_2 control and mannitol or hypertonic saline) if signs of raised ICP (see Chapter 30) and proceed to emergency surgery if necessary with the result of CT head.
- Insertion of an ICP monitor into the brain may be helpful in conditions associated with raised ICP.
- If meningitis or encephalitis is suspected, empirical antibiotics and antiviral drugs should be started pending the CSF results (see Chapter 21).
- If patient is in status epilepticus or in non-convulsive status (on EEG), load with phenytoin intravenously followed by a regular AED.
- Any obvious underlying cause if detected should be treated, for example broad-spectrum antibiotic cover (on microbiology advice) for sepsis of unknown origin; hyponatraemia or other electrolyte and acid–base disturbance; hypothermia and so on.

Remember: When approaching a comatose patient, remember to start with both assessment and management of ABC (airways, breathing and circulation).

COMPLICATIONS   These depend upon underlying cause. In general, these are a few to note:
- Airway compromise due to poor GCS.
- Progressive herniation and death due to raised ICP.

- Rapid correction of hyponatraemia leading to central pontine myelinolysis.
- Prolonged hypoglycaemia leading to irreversible brain damage.

PROGNOSIS
- Depends on underlying cause.
- Coma related to drug abuse or hypoglycaemia (if corrected quickly) has a better outcome.
- If there is no improvement, patients will need testing for brainstem death (see the following section) to decide regarding withdrawal of ventilator support.

Criteria for diagnosis of brainstem death
Prerequisites are irreversible brainstem damage, a known irreversible cause (therefore, no hypothermia, endocrine or metabolic disturbance or presence of drugs including CNS depressants or neuromuscular blockers), and no brainstem function with an unresponsive patient on ventilator (no spontaneous respiratory effort) with an adequate SBP $\geq$90 mmHg. Tests are carried out by two senior doctors on two occasions.
- Fixed and dilated pupils bilaterally.
- Absent corneal reflex.
- Absent oculocephalic and vestibulo-ocular reflex.
- Absent gag response.
- No purposeful response to painful stimuli.
- After pre-oxygenation (15 min of ventilation with 100% O_2), patient is disconnected from the ventilator to allow pCO_2 to rise to $\geq$6.65 kPa. Absence of spontaneous respiration indicates failure of respiratory centre in medulla.

DIFFERENTIAL DIAGNOSES (TABLE 31.1)

Table 31.1 Differential diagnoses for coma with points to note

Clinical conditions	Points to note
Diffuse or metabolic cause for coma	Usually equal and reactive pupils with no focal neurological deficit
Focal cause for coma: Supratentorial and infratentorial	*Supratentorial lesions*: Unilateral pupillary changes (e.g. fixed and dilated), focal motor deficit, decorticate or decerebrate posturing, asymmetry in reflexes including upgoing plantar. *Infratentorial lesions*: Coma and impairment of brainstem reflexes may occur earlier compared to supratentorial lesions
Persistent vegetative state	No awareness of self or environment with no purposeful response or movement following traumatic head injury or another cause of brain damage. Spontaneous respiration and a stable circulation present
Locked-in syndrome	Due to ventral pontine infarction and characterised by alert patients with bilateral pinpoint pupils, loss of speech and quadriplegia
Psychogenic	Catatonia, conversion reaction (inconsistent neurological findings)

32   Head injury: General approach and management

DEFINITIONS

- *Traumatic brain injury (TBI)*: An insult to the brain arising from an external mechanical force. May result from impact, acceleration–deceleration or rotational forces, blast waves or penetration of the brain by a projectile and lead to an altered state of consciousness and a permanent or temporary disturbance of cerebral function.
- *Penetrating (open) head injury*: Occurs when an object pierces the skull and breaches the dura mater.
- *Closed (blunt) head injury*: Occurs when mechanical forces are applied to the head and injure the brain, but the brain is not exposed.
- *Primary brain injury*: Damage occurring at the moment of injury due to the direct application of forces disrupting the physical integrity of the brain due to stretching, tearing and compression of tissue. Includes diffuse axonal injury, coup and contrecoup contusional injury.
- *Secondary brain injury*: Up to 40% of patients who survive the initial traumatic insult subsequently deteriorate due to secondary insults from the delayed systemic and intracranial pathophysiological consequences (Table 32.1). It is prevention of secondary brain injury that underpins emergency department and neurosurgical and intensive care management of head-injured patients.
- *Concussion*: A transient alteration of consciousness (confusion, post-traumatic amnesia (PTA) (see below) or loss of consciousness) arising as a result of a non-penetrating TBI. Normal CT imaging. A common sequelae of contact sports, players should not return to play for 1–4 weeks (depending on severity) and until symptom free.

EPIDEMIOLOGY

- Approximately 300 per 100 000 require hospital admission in the United Kingdom of whom approximately 9 per 100 000 die (5000 deaths per year).
- The incidence and relative frequencies of injury vary according to age, sex, geographical location, time of day/year and psychosocial factors.
- In the United Kingdom, road traffic accidents (RTA) account for up to 25% of TBI (60% of deaths from TBI). Other causes include falls, assault and sports injuries.
- *Highest risk groups*: Young children (0–4 years of age), young adults (15–19 years of age) and the elderly (>75 years of age). Males are twice as likely as females to sustain a TBI.

AETIOLOGY   Highly variable. Certain types of brain injury are more likely with certain mechanisms:

- *Diffuse axonal injury (DAI)*: Type of primary brain injury seen in severe closed head injuries, typically high-speed RTA, where the brain is exposed to acceleration–deceleration forces in association with rotational forces resulting in shear stresses being applied causing stretching and tearing of axons. DAI is a type of primary brain injury.
- Subdural haematoma, skull fracture and cerebral contusions (see Chapter 33); extradural haematoma (see Chapter 34).
- *Non-accidental head injury (NAHI) in infants*: Suspect if triad of injuries seen—multifocal subdural haematoma, retinal haemorrhages and encephalopathic presentation (usually with associated hypoxic–ischaemic injury on CT/MRI imaging), particularly if associated with systemic signs of inflicted injury (rib or limb fractures, burns and unexplained bruising). Most likely mechanism is shaking injury, with or without impact.

ASSOCIATIONS/RISK FACTORS

- Alcohol intoxication is associated with TBI in up to 40% of cases.
- Patients on anticoagulant or antiplatelet therapy or with a known bleeding diathesis are at increased risk of intracranial haemorrhage following TBI.

- Children with attention deficit hyperactivity disorder (ADHD) are at increased risk of TBI.
- Lower socio-economic status and educational level are associated with increased risk of TBI.

> *Remember: Spinal injuries (see Chapter 35) are strongly associated with head injury. Ensure head-injured patients are immobilised in a hard cervical collar and log-rolled until the spine is cleared clinically and/or radiologically when appropriate.*

PATHOLOGY/PATHOGENESIS   The pathological changes in the brain arising as a result of a primary brain injury depend on a number of factors, including magnitude of force of impact, intracranial vectors of transmitted force (linear and rotational), skull thickness, impact site and secondary insults (e.g. bleeding from blood vessels giving rise to haematomas or hypoxic insults leading to secondary ischaemic damage).

IMMEDIATE CLINCAL MANAGEMENT
- Stabilise airway, breathing and circulation and ensure cervical spine immobilised before attending to other injuries (including the head).
- Establish Glasgow Coma Score (see Appendix 2).

HISTORY   Establish the following from patient or witnesses:
- Mechanism and circumstances of accident. (Was there any preceding event that caused accident/fall such as a seizure?)
- Timing of accident.
- Associated injuries/symptoms, including history of headaches and vomiting.
- Duration of any loss of consciousness (LOC).
- Details of pre-hospital care—initial GCS, secondary insults (hypoxia, hypotension, cardiorespiratory arrest, blood loss and seizures).
- Posttraumatic amnesia (*PTA*):
  o It is a *transient* state of altered cognition and behaviour following concussive type injuries. The characteristic deficiencies are *anterograde amnesia* (inability to lay down new memories following TBI) and *disorientation*. Recognition is important as a marker of injury severity.
  o Patients should not be discharged until out of PTA.

EXAMINATION
- Pulse, blood pressure, respiratory rate and pattern.
- Establish GCS.
- Pupillary responses.
- Focal limb weakness.
- Signs of raised ICP (see Chapter 30).
- Record external evidence of head injury such as scalp bruising, lacerations, palpable depressed skull fracture, CSF rhinorrhoea or otorrhoea and signs of basal skull fracture (see Chapter 33).

INVESTIGATIONS
CT head: It is the investigation of choice in patients with TBI. Request immediate CT head if any of the following are present:
- GCS <13 when first assessed in ED (<14 in children and <15 in infants).
- GCS <15 when assessed in the ED 2 h after the injury.
- Suspected open, depressed or skull base fracture (see Chapter 33).
- Posttraumatic seizure.
- Focal neurological deficit.
- Amnesia of events >30 min before impact.[1]

[1]Get CT within 8 h of injury.

- More than one episode of vomiting (three or more in children).
- Tense fontanelle (infants).
- In children:
  - 'Abnormal drowsiness.'
  - Witnessed loss of consciousness >5 min.
  - Amnesia >5 min.
  - Clinical suspicion of NAHI.
  - Dangerous mechanism of injury (high-speed RTA either as pedestrian, cyclist or passenger; fall from >3 m; high-speed injury from a projectile).
- In infants:
  - Presence of bruise, swelling or laceration >5 cm on the head.
- In adults with amnesia or loss of consciousness since the injury, if
  - Coagulopathy
  - Age >65 years[1]
  - Dangerous mechanism of injury (pedestrian or cyclist struck by a motor vehicle or fall from >1 m or five stairs).[1]

MRI brain: May be helpful if additional information is required such as to assess for evidence of DAI or hypoxic–ischaemic brain injury.

Neuropsychological assessment: It is useful in the evaluation of cognitive deficits following TBI.

MANAGEMENT   The principles of management of severe head injury revolve around the prevention of secondary insults to the damaged brain (Table 32.1). Patients with GCS ≤8 require intubation and ventilation and supportive care in an Intensive Care Unit setting. They should undergo ICP monitoring to allow early identification of any rise in intracranial pressure, which should be promptly treated (see Chapter 30). Some patients with moderate head injuries felt to be at high risk of deterioration may also require ventilation and ICP monitoring. In severe head injury, the clinical aim is to maintain the cerebral perfusion pressure (CPP) between 60 and 70 mmHg at all times.

> *Remember: Exclude significant brain injury before ascribing depressed conscious level to intoxication. Alcohol intoxication is very unlikely to account for loss of more than one point on the GCS (even with severe intoxication or blood alcohol level >250 mg/ dL); therefore, do not wait for the patient to sober up, get a CT scan.*

Table 32.1 Secondary brain insults following TBI and their management

Secondary Insults	Management
Systemic	
Hypotension	Control/replace blood loss, ensure adequate fluid replacement and use pressors to maintain BP if required
Hypoxia	Protect/clear airway, optimise lung function/ventilation and ventilate if required with O_2 supplementation. Maintain PaO_2 >10 kPa
Hypercapnia	Ensure clear airway and adequate ventilation, ventilate if GCS ≤8 and monitor end tidal CO_2. Maintain $PaCO_2 = 4.5$ kPa
Anaemia	Maintain Hb >10g/dL; transfuse if required

Pyrexia	Maintain normothermia or mild hypothermia; may need active cooling, antipyretics. Stop shivering in ventilated patients with paralysing agents such as vecuronium
Systemic sepsis	Ensure prompt diagnosis and treatment of systemic sepsis. Maintain successful enteral nutrition
Hyponatraemia	Maintain Na^+ >140 mmol/L; use hypertonic saline or mannitol if required. Avoid rapid overcorrection of hyponatraemia (risk of central pontine myelinolysis)
Hyperglycaemia or hypoglycaemia	Maintain blood glucose 4–7 mmol/L
Intracranial	
Haematoma (extradural, subdural, intracerebral or intraventricular)	Prompt surgical evacuation of any haematoma causing significant mass effect (Chapters 33 and 34)
Cerebral oedema	See Chapter 30
Vascular hyperaemia/loss of autoregulation	See Chapter 30
Arterial dissection	May occur in delayed fashion. Carotid dissection (following hyperextension injury) can lead to major stroke if large vessels occluded. May require anticoagulation
Hydrocephalus	Surgical placement of external ventricular drain (EVD); in long term, it may require a VP shunt (see Chapter 37)
Seizures	Prophylactic phenytoin for 7 days to prevent early seizures; continue anticonvulsants if seizures occur
Cerebral abscess/empyema	For penetrating brain injuries: surgical debridement and broad-spectrum i.v. antibiotic cover; but no prophylactic antibiotic cover for isolated CSF leak

COMPLICATIONS

- *Epilepsy*: Risk highest in first 3 years after head injury. Highest risk is with penetrating head injury (50%).
- *CSF leak/meningitis*: CSF otorrhoea almost always resolves spontaneously. Nasal CSF leaks persisting >7 days may require surgical intervention due to risk of meningitis.
- *Hydrocephalus*: May develop months or even years after head injury. Often presents with normal pressure hydrocephalus symptoms (see Chapter 37).
- *Brain abscess* (penetrating brain injury).
- *Cranial nerve injury*: Commonly affected nerves include olfactory (I) (anosmia); optic (II) (usually damaged in foramen due to fracture, causes visual loss), abducens (VI) (skull base fractures, causes diplopia) and facial (VII) (lower motor neuron weakness, associated with skull base fracture).
- *Post-concussion symptoms*:
  - *Multifactorial aetiology*: Organic and psychosocial factors.
  - Symptoms include headache, dizziness, blurred vision, poor concentration, memory problems, mood swings, depression, irritability and loss of libido.

- *Hypopituitarism*: Affects up to 15% of patients with severe head injury. Diabetes insipidus may occur due to posterior pituitary failure.
- *Dementia pugilistica*: Dementia occurring in patients exposed to repeated head injury, for example boxers. Shares some neuropathological features of Alzheimer's disease (see Chapter 29).

PROGNOSIS   Directly related to head injury severity. Severity is determined by admission GCS (of which the motor score is the most reliable predictor), duration of PTA or by duration of LOC (Table 32.2). Mortality approaches 100% in patients with GCS 3 and bilateral fixed, dilated pupils on arrival at the ED, whereas with bilateral reactive pupils and a GCS 3, survival is 50% with approximately 10% making a good recovery. Elderly patients have a significantly poorer prognosis.

Table 32.2 Head injury severity

Severity	GCS	PTA	LOC (GCS ≤8)	Return to work for survivors (%)	Mortality (%)	Favourable outcome (%)[a]
Mild	13–15	<1 day	0–30 min	70	<1	98
Moderate	9–12	>1 to <7 days	30 min–<24 h	60	6	85
Severe	3–8	>7 days	>24 h	40	30	50

[a]Good or moderate outcome (capable of independent living, with or without some residual neurological disability) by Glasgow Outcome Scale.

Note on differential diagnoses

- Coma (see Chapter 31).
- *Subarachnoid haemorrhage*: If no definite history of trauma in a comatose patient or if symptoms preceded traumatic event (e.g. sudden headache followed by fall), consider aneurysmal SAH (see Chapter 16).
- *High cervical cord injury*: Beware of high cervical cord injury as a cause of absent motor responses when assessing GCS.

33 Head injury: Subdural haematoma, skull fractures and contusions

DEFINITION   Acute subdural haematoma (ASDH) refers to presence of fresh blood in the subdural space usually due to trauma. Most chronic subdural haematomas (CSDH) follow an ASDH and mainly affect the elderly population.

EPIDEMIOLOGY   Incidence of CSDH is highest in the elderly, with a peak incidence in the eighth decade.

AETIOLOGY   ASDH usually occurs following trauma leading to head injury, for example road traffic accidents. Patients receiving anticoagulation therapy can sustain an ASDH even with minimal trauma.
CSDH in the elderly follows an untreated ASDH or a traumatic subdural CSF effusion, typically in patients with a degree of cerebral atrophy and can also occur in the context of *minimal trauma*. There may not be a history of trauma in up to 50% of patients with CSDH. Spontaneous subdural haematoma (acute or chronic), unrelated to trauma, can be due to hypertension, arteriovenous malformations, aneurysm, infection and neoplasm.

Remember: CSDH can occur in the elderly in the context of minimal trauma to head.

ASSOCIATIONS/RISK FACTORS   Apart from blunt trauma and age >60 years, risk factors for CSDH include coagulopathies, for example related to liver disease, iatrogenic therapeutic anticoagulation or alcohol abuse; recurrent falls, for example in patients with dementia syndromes or with hemiplegia as a result of previous stroke; any condition causing significant cerebral atrophy (alcoholism, dementia etc.) and patients with shunts, for example a ventriculoperitoneal shunt for normal pressure hydrocephalus (see Chapter 37). Anticoagulation therapy also increases the risk for an ASDH.

PATHOLOGY/PATHOGENESIS   ASDH are usually associated with severe impact damage and primary injury to the brain. It can arise either from oozing/accumulation around an area of laceration to the brain parenchyma, usually in the frontal or temporal region or due to rupture of a bridging vein from acceleration–deceleration during rapid movement of the head. In the latter case, particularly in cases where the bridging veins are stretched due to cerebral atrophy and therefore more susceptible to injury with lesser degrees of force, the underlying brain injury may be mild and patients' presentation may mimic that of an acute extradural haematoma with a lucid interval followed by a rapid deterioration. Rupture of a cortical artery may also result in ASDH.

HISTORY   ASDH, usually subsequent to trauma, for example falls or road traffic accidents, can mimic extradural haematoma in its presentation with a lucid interval prior to deterioration. In younger patients, ASDH is typically associated with high-velocity blunt head trauma and patients are often comatose from the outset. It can also present with a more gradual deterioration in GCS with haematoma expansion, headache, nausea and vomiting. Seizures may occur in the posttraumatic period.
Diagnosis of CSDH on average occurs 4–5 weeks following trauma. CSDH patients can present insidiously with symptoms mimicking TIA, headaches, confusion and cognitive decline, nausea and vomiting, change in personality and episodes of speech arrest or dysfunction (with dominant hemisphere lesions). Fluctuation in symptoms may be marked. Patients may complain of weakness, usually contralateral to the side of the haematoma.

Remember: ASDH is arbitrarily defined as presenting 1–3 days after injury, subacute SDH as presenting 4 days to 3 weeks after injury and CSDH as presenting more than 3 weeks after the injury.

EXAMINATION   Findings associated with ASDH may include the following (also see Chapter 30):
- Deterioration in conscious level (GCS) as above.
- Dilated, unreactive pupil ipsilateral to the haematoma.
- Focal neurological deficits, for example dysphasia and sensory disturbance, and long tract signs, for example hemiparesis usually contralateral to the side of haematoma.

Findings associated with CSDH may include the following:
- Reduced level of consciousness, focal neurological deficits as above, reflex asymmetry and gait disturbance.
- Evidence of dysphasia (may be fluctuating) with dominant hemisphere collection.
- Reduced scores on mini-mental state examination in patients with CSDH and associated cognitive decline (a treatable cause of dementia).

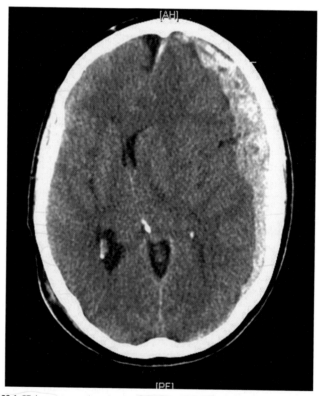

Figure 33.1 CT demonstrates a large hyperdense ASDH over frontal, temporal and parietal convexity with significant mass effect, i.e. midline shift and effacement of ventricles. Note the characteristic crescentic shape of the clot.

Remember: Hemiparesis may occur ipsilateral to the side of the haematoma if contra-lateral cerebral peduncle is compressed against the edge of the tentorium cerebelli, the so-called 'Kernohan notch phenomenon'.

INVESTIGATIONS

- *Blood tests:* FBC, U & E (particularly sodium level check) and clotting parameters (correct any coagulopathy).
- *CT:* Crescentic blood collection (concave towards brain surface) with varying attenuation depending on the clot age. An acute collection (Figure 33.1) will be hyperdense, subacute isodense (Figure 33.2) and chronic hypodense (similar to the density of CSF) (Figure 33.3) in comparison to the density of brain parenchyma. Some collections may have mixed density, for example due to a new haemorrhage into an old collection, the so-called 'acute on chronic SDH'.

Remember: Concave (crescentic shape) towards brain surface on CT for SDH as opposed to convex (biconvex shape) for EDH.

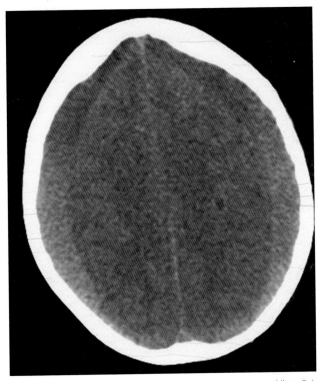

Figure 33.2 CT demonstrates mixed density bilateral SDH. The posterior component bilaterally is subacute as is isodense with the brain parenchyma. Note that these are easy to miss on the scan!

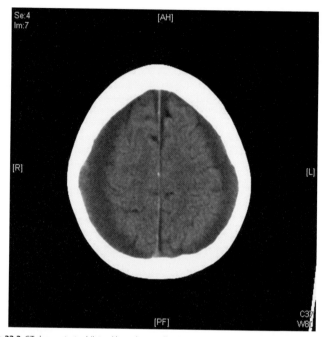

Figure 33.3 CT demonstrates bilateral hypodense collection concave towards the brain's surface, characteristic of CSDH.

MANAGEMENT Symptomatic ASDH greater than 1 cm at the thickest point with associated mass effect should be considered for rapid surgical evacuation via a craniotomy. An asymptomatic smaller SDH may be managed conservatively with careful monitoring of patient's neurological status and surveillance of size of collection using CT.

Symptomatic CSDH with mass effect is generally managed using two burr holes and irrigation with warm saline until clear. Typically dark fluid resembling 'motor oil' is evacuated with subsequent placement of a subdural drain (for 24–48 h) to decrease the risk of reaccumulation. Recurrence following evacuation occurs in 5–30% of patients.

COMPLICATIONS Untreated both acute and chronic SDH can lead to significant morbidity and mortality from both mass effect and seizures.

Complications related to surgical treatment may include seizures, recurrence, tension pneumocephalus (air within subdural space), subdural empyema, intracerebral haemorrhage and death.

PROGNOSIS Mortality rates can vary for ASDH between 50% and 90%, with mortality being higher in patients over 40 years of age, those with a poor initial or postresuscitation GCS and those with associated ischaemic or diffuse axonal brain injury. Thirty day mortality associated with surgical treatment of CSDH varies between 0% and 8%.

DIFFERENTIAL DIAGNOSIS See Table 34.1.

Other Conditions of note (Table 33.1)

Table 33.1 Other conditions of note related to trauma and head injury

Clinical conditions	Points to note
Haemorrhagic contusion or traumatic intracerebral haematoma (Figure 33.4)	Occurs following head trauma due to sudden deceleration and impact of brain against bony prominences, for example in basal frontal and temporal areas in coup (lying immediately under the point of impact) or contrecoup (opposite the point of impact, for example frontal contusions arising from a blow to the occiput) fashion
	These may enlarge and blossom with time
	Admit patients for close neurological observations
	Surgical intervention if significant mass effect and deterioration in GCS
Depressed skull fracture (Figure 33.5)	Can be classified as closed (simple) or open (compound) fractures (if in communication with an overlying scalp laceration)
	A simple linear fracture without displacement does not require surgical intervention
	An open depressed fracture needs repair and debridement of overlying skin laceration and elevation of fracture surgically if depression is greater than thickness of skull or if associated with CSF leak or neurological deficit
	Closed depressed fractures may be managed conservatively if the degree of depression is cosmetically acceptable (discuss with a neurosurgeon)
	Posttraumatic seizures can occur
Basal skull fracture[a]	Extension of fractures from cranial vault
	Signs: Anosmia, VIIth and VIIIth nerve injury (temporal bone fracture), CSF rhinorrhoea or otorrhoea, Battle's sign (mastoid bruising), haemotympanum and periorbital bruising
	CT (bone windows with thin cuts) can be used for diagnosis; also look for pneumocephalus
	Usually managed conservatively
Penetrating brain injury	If low velocity, it may not be associated with loss of consciousness
	Neurological deficit relates to focal area of brain damage
	Surgical debridement and antibiotic therapy are required
	Beware that cases where the penetrating implement has been removed, neuroradiological imaging is required to rule out any underlying brain or vascular injury

[a]*Remember: Blind placement of an NG tube is contraindicated in cases of suspected basal skull fracture, as it can be passed intracranially if cribriform plate is fractured.*

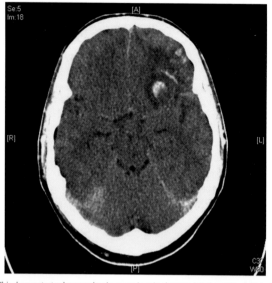

Figure 33.4 This demonstrates haemorrhagic contusions in characteristic basal frontal lobe location with associated pericontusional oedema.

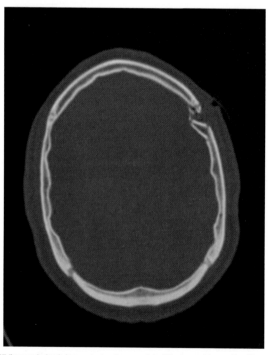

Figure 33.5 CT (bone window) demonstrates depressed skull fracture with associated intracranial air. This needed surgical elevation.

34 Head injury: Extradural haematoma

DEFINITION   Traumatic accumulation of blood/haematoma between the 'stripped-off' dura and the inner table of the skull.

EPIDEMIOLOGY
- One per cent of head trauma admissions; male:female = 4:1.
- Mainly occurs in young adults; rare before 2 or after 60 years of age (as dura is more adherent to the bone at the extremes of the age).

AETIOLOGY   Traumatic injury to the head, for example in the setting of road traffic accidents or a focussed blow to the head such as with a baseball bat/boxing.

ASSOCIATIONS/RISK FACTORS
- Up to 85% have associated skull fracture due to traumatic head injury.
- Up to 20% can have associated acute subdural haematoma.
- Age (peak age between 10 and 30 years with patients younger than 20 years of age accounting for 60% of EDHs).

PATHOLOGY/PATHOGENESIS
- Majority of EDHs (85%) are due to arterial bleeding and most commonly in the temporoparietal region.
- Damage of the middle meningeal artery by temporoparietal skull fracture (centred around Pterion) due to trauma leading to arterial bleeding and dissection of dura from inner table of the skull.
- Remainder are due to bleeding from dural sinus or diploic vein.

HISTORY
- *'Textbook/classical' presentation (<10–27% of cases)*:
  - Brief posttraumatic loss of consciousness.
  - Followed by recovery and a 'lucid interval' (between initial trauma and subsequent neurological deterioration).
  - Leading to neurological decline with decreasing GCS.
  - Finally, if untreated, death due to 'herniation' (usually uncal).
- *Other presenting complaints*: Headache, vomiting and seizures.
- Deterioration usually over 'few' hours.

> *Remember: Only up to one-third of cases with EDHs have the characteristic lucid interval before deterioration; therefore, even in the absence of the 'textbook presentation', EDHs must be suspected and ruled out in patients presenting with decreased GCS, headache, vomiting, seizure or focal neurological deficits following head trauma.*

EXAMINATION
- Scalp laceration or bony step-off in the area of injury, otorrhoea, rhinorrhoea and haemotympanum.
- Decreased or fluctuating GCS with or without focal neurological deficits.
- Ipsilateral pupillary dilatation (due to increased ICP and compression of oculomotor nerve) (see Chapter 30).
- Contralateral hemiparesis (due to compression of ipsilateral cerebral peduncle).
- *Ipsilateral hemiplegia or hemiparesis*: Can occur as a 'false localising sign' due to compression of contralateral cerebral peduncle against the tentorial edge (the so-called 'Kernohan' notch phenomenon).

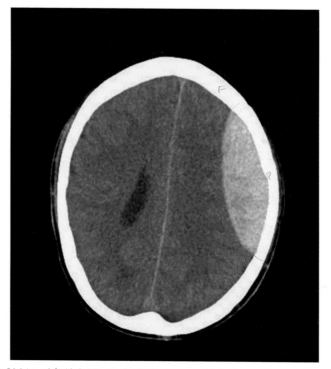

Figure 34.1 Large left-sided acute extradural haematoma associated with mass effect and effacement of the ipsilateral lateral ventricle. Note the characteristic biconvex 'lens' shape of the clot.

- In later stages due to progression and herniation:
  - ○ Coma and decerebrate rigidity.
  - ○ Cushing response (hypertension, bradycardia and respiratory irregularity) and death.

INVESTIGATION
- *Plain skull X-ray*: May show skull fracture.
- *Unenhanced head CT scan* (Figure 34.1): Compare with acute subdural haematoma (Table 34.1) (also see Chapter 33)—
  - ○ Done urgently as a procedure of choice for diagnosis.
  - ○ Blood appears as high density (white).
  - ○ Biconvex (lenticular) shape (adjacent to skull).
  - ○ Uniform density with sharply defined edges.
  - ○ Usually confined to small segment of calvaria.
  - ○ Blood in EDH does not cross suture lines (dura is attached more firmly to skull at sutures).
  - ○ Allows assessment of associated mass effect and other intracranial injuries/haematoma.
- *Cervical spine evaluation*: Exclude any associated neck injury using plain films and CT of cervical spine if needed.

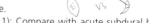

Remember: Urgent/immediate unenhanced head CT scan is the procedure of choice to confirm or exclude EDH in a patient who has sustained head trauma.

elaborate bld
glucose, fluids, O₂
hypothermia
mannitol
intubate/ventilate
CSF drain

MANAGEMENT

- *Medical*:
  - ○ Manage airway, breathing and circulation.
  - ○ General management of head trauma and increased ICP (see Chapter 30).
  - ○ Small asymptomatic EDHs can be followed up with serial CT.
- *Surgical*:
  - ○ For any symptomatic EDH.
  - ○ Acute asymptomatic EDH >30 mL volume or with >5 mm of midline shift.
  - ○ Urgent craniotomy and evacuation of the clot with haemostasis.

> *Remember: EDH in majority of cases requires urgent surgery and therefore all cases with EDH should be referred immediately to the regional neurosurgical centre.*

COMPLICATIONS

- Permanent neurological deficits.
- Death (due to respiratory arrest from uncal herniation and injury to midbrain).

PROGNOSIS

- About 5–10% mortality (if optimal diagnosis and prompt treatment within 'few' hours).
- Underlying brain parenchyma is relatively intact if EDH is treated promptly.
- Higher morbidity and mortality with delayed treatment.

> *Remember: Prompt diagnosis and urgent surgical treatment of EDH significantly reduces the mortality associated with this condition.*

DIFFERENTIAL DIAGNOSES

Table 34.1 Differential diagnoses with appropriate investigations

Clinical condition	How to exclude it? (investigations to do)
Acute subdural haematoma (ASDH) (Chapter 33)	*CT head*: Hyperdense collection (clot), *crescentic shaped and crosses suture lines*. Remember these can coexist with EDH
Subarachnoid haemorrhage (SAH) (Chapter 16)	*CT Head*: Hyperdense blood within subarachnoid spaces; Lumbar puncture looking for xanthochromia if CT head is negative and there is a high index of clinical suspicion for SAH
Intracerebral haemorrhage (ICH) (Chapter 15)	Relevant history regarding trauma, hypertension, coagulopathies, vascular malformations, alcohol and recreational drugs. *CT Head*: Blood as high density within brain parenchyma. Note trauma can cause all of the above, i.e. EDH, ASDH, SAH and ICH

35 Spinal injuries and spinal cord syndromes

DEFINITION

Complete spinal cord injury (SCI): Complete loss of all sensory and motor (upper motor neuron lesion) function below lesion.

Incomplete spinal cord injury: Some preservation of motor and/or sensory function. Specific subtypes of incomplete lesions are shown in Table 35.1.

Table 35.1 Incomplete spinal cord injury syndromes

Cord syndrome	Key features	Causes
Central cord syndrome	Weakness of upper extremities > lower extremities (first to recover). Variable sensory deficit. Sphincter disturbance	Acute hyperextension injury on background of cervical stenosis
Anterior cord syndrome	Paraplegia (tetraplegia if above C7) and dissociated sensory loss (loss of pain and temperature and preservation of other sensory modalities) below the lesion	Cord infarction in anterior spinal artery territory. Anterior cord compression by traumatic disc herniation or fracture fragment
Brown–Sequard syndrome	Ipsilateral paralysis and spasticity and loss of proprioception and vibration (posterior column function); contralateral loss of pain and temperature (spinothalamic tract) starting 1–2 levels below lesion. Loss of all ipsilateral modalities at the level of lesion	Spinal cord hemisection (penetrating trauma), lateral cord compression from disc herniation, tumour or haematoma
Posterior cord syndrome (rare)	Pain and dysaesthesia (burning) in cape distribution (neck, upper arms and torso); posterior column (proprioception and vibration) dysfunction and preserved pain and temperature sensation. Mild upper extremity paresis. No or few long tract signs	Hyperextension injury especially with posterior arch fractures, penetrating trauma or posterior spinal artery infarction

SCIWORA (*spinal cord injury without radiographic abnormality*): Seen in children. Traumatic ligamentous/soft tissue spinal column injury causes instability. Assess with MRI.

EPIDEMIOLOGY   Approximately 40% motor vehicle accidents; 40% sports injuries/assaults and 20% falls. The cervical spine is the most commonly injured.

AETIOLOGY   Usually associated with unstable fractures of the spinal column. See below for details of common spinal fractures.

ASSOCIATIONS/RISK FACTORS

Head injury: Regard anyone with a significant head injury as having a possible unstable spinal column injury.

Diving into shallow water (*or other axial loading*).

Leisure and sporting activities: High-risk activities include horse riding, rugby, American football and trampolining.

Loss of bone strength: Rheumatoid arthritis, osteoporosis and bone tumours including metastases. These can result in spinal cord injury with trivial trauma.

Coagulopathy: Patients with bleeding disorders or on anticoagulant therapy may develop epidural (most common), subdural or intramedullary haematomas, either spontaneously or following trivial trauma. Be suspicious if patient has a progressive neurological deficit.

Remember the association between head injury and cervical spine injury and therefore the need to immobilise and log-roll these patients, until spinal injury is excluded clinically and/or radiologically as appropriate.

PATHOLOGY/PATHOGENESIS

Spinal shock: Refers to the transient loss of all neurological function below the level of the spinal cord injury causing a flaccid paralysis and arreflexia that usually persists for around 2 weeks after the injury. Following resolution, an upper motor neuron deficit develops with exaggerated reflexes and extensor plantar reflexes, due to loss of descending inhibition of spinal cord reflex arcs.

Remember: Spinal shock is also sometimes used to refer to the hypotension that accompanies acute cervical/upper thoracic spinal cord injury caused by abrupt loss of sympathetic tone, with unopposed parasympathetic activity, and impaired venous return (loss of muscle pump due to flaccid paralysis) resulting in relative hypovolaemia. It is important that this is actively managed as it may exacerbate cord injury due to hypoperfusion.

HISTORY

Remember: The initial management of traumatic spinal cord injury should follow ATLS guidelines.

The clinical history should include a detailed description of the mechanism of injury as this may inform the nature of the injury to the spinal column (e.g. hyperflexion, hyperextension, axial compression and distraction). The presence of *focal neck* or *back pain* may assist in injury localisation. The immediate neurological symptoms should be recorded, and history of a progressive neurological deficit should raise suspicion of an evolving haematoma or severe instability with ongoing cord compromise. The history should include any risk factors identified above that may predispose to traumatic SCI.

EXAMINATION In fully conscious, neurologically intact, *non-intoxicated* trauma patients, the posterior cervical spine should be palpated for any focal tenderness. If pain free and without high-risk factors for spinal injury (see below), they should be asked to turn their head 45 degrees to each side; if this does not cause significant pain, a fracture can be clinically ruled out.

Log-roll the patient and palpate the spine for any 'step' or focal tenderness and look for bruising and also perform a rectal exam to assess anal sphincter contraction. Palpate the abdomen and feel for a full bladder (urinary retention). Perform a full neurological examination including motor and sensory (pain, light touch and proprioception) function, reflexes (tendon jerks initially absent in cord injury) including abdominal and sacral reflexes and observe for any sign of autonomic dysfunction such as incontinence or priapism.

> *Remember: A spinal fracture cannot be clinically excluded in an intoxicated patient or a patient with a distracting injury; in these cases, appropriate imaging of spine (initially plain X-rays and then CT (if needed)) should be obtained to exclude a fracture (see below).*

INVESTIGATIONS The neck should be imaged in any blunt trauma patient with a depressed level of consciousness, abnormal vital signs, neurological symptoms or signs, severe neck pain (>7/10) or tenderness, a low-risk mechanism but restricted/painful movement, or with neck pain or tenderness and a visible injury above the clavicle or severely painful thoracic trauma and a high risk mechanism of injury (fall >1 m or five stairs, axial loading injury (e.g. diving), motor vehicle accident (>60 mph combined speed or rollover), bicycle collision, age >65 years and distracting injury).

Plain X-rays: Should include three views (AP, lateral and open mouth odontoid views) and show 0/C1 and C7/T1 levels (ask for 'swimmers view' if cannot see C7/T1). Films of the thoracic and lumbar spine should be used to clear these areas in unconscious/ventilated patients and in those with an abnormal clinical examination including focal tenderness.

CT: Required in any patient with abnormal/inadequate plain films. In the cervical spine, it is the preferred imaging modality in patients with: GCS <13 or intubated, new neurological signs, severe neck pain or known spinal disease (e.g. ankylosing spondylitis and rheumatoid arthritis), and those requiring a CT head.

MRI: Use in patients with suspected cord pathology without history of trauma. In trauma, it should always be used in conjunction with CT and is indicated in any patient with focal neurological signs, those at risk of vertebral artery injury (e.g. posterior circulation syndrome) or those with a normal CT but severe neck pain or restricted movement.

Dynamic plain X-rays: Flexion extension views may be required for patient with possible occult ligamentous instability without significant bony injury.

Bone scan: Can be used to differentiate recent from old injuries.

MANAGEMENT
Fracture: Patients with possible spinal injury are initially managed in the field with immobilisation on a spinal board, hard cervical collar and sandbags either side of the head until significant injury is excluded.

> *Remember: For spinal fractures, the principles of management are reduction of any deformity (e.g. skull traction to reduce facet dislocation) and immobilisation (either by hard collar, halo vest or surgical internal fixation) for potentially unstable injuries.*

Unstable thoracolumbar fractures can be managed with bed rest with log-rolling pending any definitive surgical treatment.

Acute spinal cord injury: Medical management includes ensuring adequate blood pressure (with pressors if necessary) and oxygenation; NG tube (decompress abdomen); urinary catheter (decompress bladder) and DVT thromboprophylaxis. Patients with incomplete cord injury and evidence of ongoing cord compression should undergo urgent decompressive surgery (e.g. fracture reduction, evacuation of haematoma and excision of traumatic disc prolapse). In patients with non-traumatic cord injury, the underlying cause should be addressed (e.g. surgical resection of compressive tumour; foramen magnum decompression for Chiari I malformation with syringomyelia).

COMPLICATIONS
Autonomic dysreflexia: It is a serious, life-threatening condition usually arising in patients with cervical and upper thoracic (above T6) cord injury. Activation of afferent autonomic

pathways typically by urinary retention or faecal impaction (but can be noxious stimuli below lesion such as in-growing toenails, UTI, pressure sores, burns, tight or restrictive clothing, labour and delivery) causes reflex discharge from splanchnic sympathetic outflow (T5/L2) resulting in massive sympathetic discharge causing severe hypertension, pounding headache, and vascoconstriction (below the lesion). The normal homeostatic feedback is interrupted by the lesion resulting in increased parasympathetic output causing bradycardia and flushing, profuse sweating and piloerection (above the lesion). Treatment: Sit up to encourage orthostatic hypotension and lower ICP, identify and treat possible causes (e.g. urinary catheterisation and loosen tight clothing) and severe hypertension may require specific medical treatment.

Remember: Sweating with pounding headache in a spinal cord-injured patient should prompt immediate investigation for autonomic dysreflexia.

Respiratory infections: Higher lesion weakness of intercostal and abdominal muscles results in a poor cough with retained secretions and an increased risk of infection.
Prevention/treatment: Physiotherapy, mini-tracheostomy to facilitate secretion clearance and ventilatory support.
Pressure sores: Meticulous care of insensate pressure areas is required.
DVT/PE: High-risk group, ensure prophylactic low molecular weight heparin administered for first 3 months after injury.
Osteoporosis: Can result in pathological fractures. Prevent with bisphosphonates.
Heterotopic ossification: Causes ossification of soft tissues around joints resulting in loss of movement, seen on X-ray and associated with elevated serum alkaline phosphatase. Bisphosphonates or non-steroidal anti-inflammatory drugs (e.g. indomethacin) used as prophylaxis.
Scoliosis: Young children with SCI at greatest risk. Can lead to respiratory compromise.
Urinary tract sepsis and renal impairment: Common source of sepsis. Use intermittent self-catheterisation to reduce risk.
Spasticity and contractures: Muscular spasms may be either spontaneous or provoked by neurogenic irritation such as a full bladder, or bowel, or infection; treat with antispasmodics or treat the precipitating cause. Contractures (which may otherwise prevent successful rehabilitation) should be prevented with physiotherapy, antispasmodics such as baclofen and injection of botulinum toxin into affected muscles.
Syringomyelia: A late complication that can occur many years later, the syrinx (a CSF-filled cavity within the spinal cord) usually forms at the level of trauma due to scarring of the arachnoid membrane around cord causing obstruction of CSF flow. Presentation is with new onset of neurological signs: a *dissociated* (pain and temperature affected initially as decussating, more centrally located spinothalamic fibres are more vulnerable to damage from centrally expanding syrinx) sensory loss, motor deficit and neuropathic pain (ascending above the level of the original lesion). Diagnosis is with MRI to demonstrate CSF accumulation within the spinal cord.
Suicide: Accounts for 10% of mortality of SCI patients.

Remember: Sensory loss in syringomyelia is dissociated as initially pain and temperature sensation (spinothalamic tract) is affected with preservation of joint position and vibration sense (dorsal column).

PROGNOSIS   Recovery of function is greatest within the first 6 months after injury, the majority of neurological deficits persisting longer than 12 months after injury will not recover.

Mortality is highest within the first 2 years of injury. After 2 years, survival is influenced by injury level (C1–C4 < C5–C8 < paraplegia), ventilator dependence, the presence of a gastrostomy, complete or incomplete SCI, associated brain injury and the patient age at the time of injury. A 30-year-old ventilator-dependent tetraplegic patient surviving more that 2 years has an actuarial life expectancy of 18 years. Pneumonia is the most common single cause of death.

DIFFERENTIAL DIAGNOSES (TABLES 35.1 AND 35.2)

Notes on common cervical spine fractures

- Common injuries include fracture–dislocation, fracture and dislocation.
- *Jefferson's fracture* (Figure 35.1): Fracture through anterior and posterior arch of the atlas (four-point burst fracture) related to axial loading, may be unstable if transverse ligament is compromised. Usually managed conservatively with a cervical collar (cervical immobilization) for approximately 12 weeks.
- *Hangman's fracture* (Figure 35.2): Defined as fracture bilaterally through the pars inter-articularis of C2 with associated anterior subluxation of C2 on C3. Occurs due to a combination of hyperextension and axial loading. Fracture tends to be stable and patients usually do not usually have a neurological deficit. Most patients again can be managed conservatively in a cervical collar (cervical immobilization) for 8–14 weeks. Surgical treatment may be required in a few patients, for example anterior C2–C3 discectomy and fusion.

Table 35.2 Differential diagnoses

Clinical conditions	Points to note
Spinal cord stroke	Abrupt onset of severe deficit with associated spinal pain
Spinal arteriovenous malformation/ arteriovenous fistula	Subacute or chronic onset of symptoms that may fluctuate; can also present with acute subarachnoid haemorrhage with abrupt severe back pain
Malignancy (spinal cord) (see Appendix 3 & 4 and Chapters 9 and 23)	Usually subacute or chronic, progressive onset of cord dysfunction. Pain is often the first symptom in patients with spinal extradural metastases and can be radicular or referred, often worse with recumbency (at night). Common malignancies involving spinal column are lymphoma, lung, breast, prostate and those from GI tract. Diagnosis not to be missed!
Transverse myelitis (Chapter 18)	Inflammatory process affecting the spinal cord (e.g. due to multiple sclerosis or viral infection); symptoms may include motor, sensory and sphincter deficits. Can lead to complete paralysis and sensory loss below the level of the lesion
Guillan–Barre syndrome (Chapter 24)	An acute, inflammatory, demyelinating, predominantly motor polyradiculoneuropathy. Can cause mild to severe weakness, mild sensory symptoms and absence of reflexes with dysfunction of autonomic nervous system. Measure vital capacity regularly in these patients as may need ventilation
Conversion disorder	A diagnosis of exclusion. Suspect if incongruent neurological signs, normal reflexes and normal MR imaging

See Tables 9.1 and 26.1.

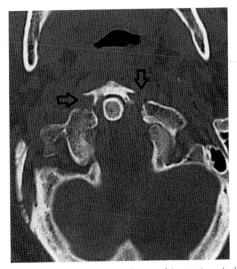

Figure 35.1 Axial CT of cervical spine demonstrating a fracture of the anterior arch of C1 (atlas)—Jefferson's fracture.

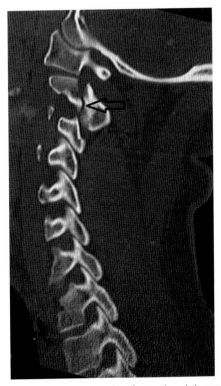

Figure 35.2 Sagittal CT of cervical spine demonstrating a fracture through the pars interarticularis of C2.

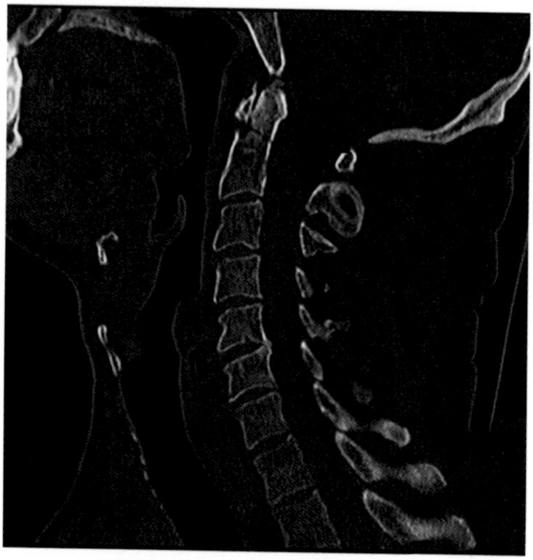

Figure 35.3 Sagittal CT of cervical spine demonstrating a type 2 fracture of odontoid peg (C2).

- *Odontoid peg fracture* (Figure 35.3): Usually seen in elderly population after a fall leading to head injury and subsequent trauma to neck (commonly in the setting of a flexion injury). Can be associated with neck pain (including on palpation over spine) and limitation of range of neck movement. Three different subtypes: Type I—fracture through tip of the dens, Type 2—fracture at the base of the dens—and Type 3—fracture goes through body of C2. Treatment options include immobilisation using a cervical collar or halo vest (10–12 weeks) or surgery (atlantoaxial fusion or anterior odontoid screw fixation).

36   CNS neoplasia

PATHOLOGY   Cerebral metastases are the most common tumour in the CNS. Neuroepithelial tumours comprise the majority of 'primary' brain tumours and are detailed in Appendix 1. Tumours can also arise from the meninges, the cranial and spinal nerves, and from the other cell types found in the CNS and are detailed in Appendix 2.

> *Remember: Cerebral metastases are the most common tumours in the CNS.*

HISTORY AND EXAMINATION   For presentation of specific tumour types, please see Appendices 1 and 2.

The following are the key general modes of presentation of CNS tumours:
- *Progressive focal neurological deficit*:
  - Due to local mass effect, compression or invasion of surrounding neural structures.
  - Most common is a progressive motor deficit.

> *Remember: Think carefully about the function of the different parts of the brain (see Chapter 3), and ask patients (or their carers) about any specific neurological deficits (including cognitive problems). Localise tumour on the basis of which functions have been lost, for example a Gerstmann's syndrome may be due to a dominant parietal lobe tumour.*

- *Symptoms and signs of raised intracranial pressure*:
  - See Chapter 30.
  - Headaches, mental status changes and papilloedema.
- *Seizures*:
  - See Chapter 17.
  - Any new onset of seizure disorder in an adult should prompt detailed investigations for an underlying tumour.
  - Seizures rarely occur in posterior fossa tumours.
- *Hydrocephalus*:
  - See Chapter 37.
  - *Obstructive*: Due to compression or obstruction of ventricular CSF pathways by tumour mass.
  - *Communicating*: Due to meningeal infiltration impairing CSF absorption.
- *Endocrine disturbance*:
  - Tumours in and around the pituitary fossa may cause hypopituitarism (see Appendix 2) due to local mass effect disturbing pituitary function.
  - Some pituitary tumours may actively secrete hormones (see Appendix 2).

INVESTIGATIONS

CT head +/– contrast: Good initial investigation in patient with acute presentation, particularly if depressed level of consciousness or seizure. Will readily identify tumour-related complications such as acute obstructive hydrocephalus or intra-tumoural haemorrhage (Figure 36.1).

MRI brain and spine +/– gadolinium contrast: Gold standard investigation for tumour localisation, radiological diagnosis and identification of metastatic disease (Figure 36.2). If a brain tumour is identified, spinal MRI should routinely be undertaken to identify spinal drop metastases. Specialised sequences such as MR tractography may allow relationship

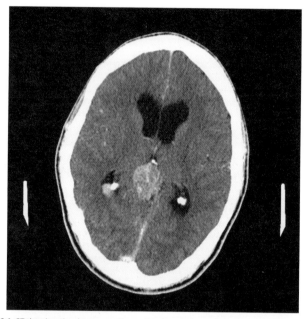

Figure 36.1 CT showing pineal tumour with associated acute obstructive hydrocephalus.

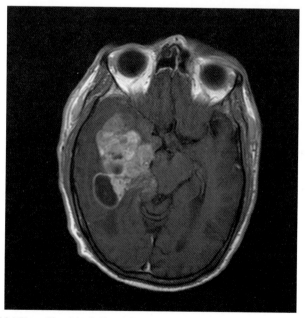

Figure 36.2 MRI scan (T1 weighted with gadolinium) showing a partly cystic partly solid enhancing mass lesion consistent with malignant glioblastoma multiforme in right temporal lobe associated with mass effect and uncal herniation.

between tumour and white matter tracts to be determined for surgical planning and MR spectroscopy may facilitate differentiation of tumour types and mimics (see below).

Other:

- *CT chest abdomen and pelvis*: Required whenever the radiological diagnosis could include CNS metastasis. Similarly, mammography may be required in selected cases.
- *Cerebral angiography*: Not usually diagnostically helpful, but may identify tumours suitable for preoperative embolisation if tumour felt likely to be vascular in nature.
- *Haematological and CSF investigations*: For certain tumour types such as pituitary tumours and Germ cell tumours, specific haematological or CSF investigations may be required (see Appendix 2).

MANAGEMENT   Patients with tumours that exert significant mass effect may require *steroid therapy* (*dexamethasone*) to help control symptoms and facilitate surgery. The exception is patients in whom a diagnosis of cerebral lymphoma is suspected, where steroid therapy should be deferred until a tumour biopsy has been performed.

The specific management of CNS tumours depends on the tumour type (see Appendices 1 and 2 for details); in some cases, the diagnosis may be radiologically obvious; in other cases, a biopsy may be required to confirm diagnosis. In cases where tumour removal is required regardless of diagnosis, for example due to symptomatic local mass effect, biopsy may be omitted in favour of tumour resection. Treatment options for other tumours include combinations of either surgery or stereotactic radiosurgery (the 'gamma knife') and/or radiotherapy and/or chemotherapy and are usually determined in the setting of a multidisciplinary team meeting. Some pituitary tumours may respond to endocrine therapy. Some benign/low-grade tumours may be managed with radiological surveillance only if small and asymptomatic.

In patients presenting with seizures, anticonvulsants may be required.

Once tumours have undergone definitive treatment, most patients will require ongoing radiological surveillance to monitor for recurrence.

COMPLICATIONS

- Progressive neurological deficit.
- Seizures.
- Hydrocephalus.
- Intratumoural haemorrhage with abrupt neurological deterioration.
- Metastasis within the CNS (spread outside the CNS is very rare).

PROGNOSIS   Long-term survival is primarily determined by the tumour type; completely resected benign and low-grade tumours may be cured. Extent of surgical resection and, if appropriate, adjuvant therapy also influence survival. Age and performance status are also important predictors of survival. The survival for high-grade malignant gliomas (glioblastoma multiforme) is dismal, with median survival rates less than 1 year even with maximal therapy.

DIFFERENTIAL DIAGNOSES   Many tumour types may be readily diagnosed on MRI imaging. Ring-enhancing parenchymal brain lesions have a number of important differential diagnoses that are detailed below (Table 36.1).

Table 36.1 Differential diagnoses for ring-enhancing parenchymal mass lesions

Clinical conditions	Points to note
Cerebral abscess (Chapter 22)	Assess for other clinical and laboratory evidence of infection. The history of any progressive deficit is usually rapid compared to that for tumour. The key investigation is diffusion-weighted MR imaging as cerebral abscess cavities have restricted diffusion whereas tumours usually do not. If in doubt, a biopsy should be urgently undertaken

(continued)

Table 36.1 (*Continued*)

Clinical conditions	Points to note
Toxoplasmosis (Chapter 22)	Usually multiple small ring-enhancing lesions with predilection for the basal ganglia and exerting little mass effect. Patients often have cerebral atrophy. Associated with HIV infection and immunosuppression
Radiation necrosis	An important differential in patients suspected of harbouring a recurrent parenchymal brain tumour who have undergone previous radiotherapy. Careful MR evaluation including MR spectroscopy may help differentiate. Biopsy or surveillance imaging may be needed
Resolving haematoma	On MR look for blood products on gradient echo sequence, a continuous ring of hypointensity is seen in haematoma. Often a follow-up scan is required a few weeks later to ensure the bleed did not arise from an underlying tumour
Stroke (Chapter 14)	An infarct may be ring enhancing. Look to see if it conforms to a vascular territory or in the case of venous infarction, whether the nearby venous sinuses are occluded
Trauma	A careful history may identify an episode of trauma. Again, a delayed follow-up scan may be required to rule out an underlying tumour
Demyelinating lesions (Chapter 18)	Tumefactive demyelinating lesions may mimic tumours. MR spectroscopy may show a high glutamate/glutamine peak, not usually seen in malignant CNS neoplasms. CSF analysis for oligoclonal bands may be required. In rare cases, biopsy may be necessary to confirm the diagnosis

37   Hydrocephalus

DEFINITION   The abnormal accumulation of CSF within the ventricles of the brain, due to a disturbance of CSF flow, absorption or (rarely) excessive production.

EPIDEMIOLOGY   Estimated prevalence is 1–1.5%. Incidence of congenital hydrocephalus is approximately 1/1000 live births, higher in third world.

AETIOLOGY
Obstructive hydrocephalus:
- Due to blockage to CSF flow within the ventricular system.
- Results in dilatation of ventricles proximal to block, for example in congenital aqueduct stenosis, the lateral and third ventricles only are enlarged.
- Any intracranial mass lesion that compresses or occludes the ventricular system can cause obstructive hydrocephalus, including tumours, haematomas and cerebral abscesses.
- Congenital causes also include Chiari I and Chiari II malformations (the latter associated with spina bifida (myelomeningocele) and Dandy Walker syndrome (atresia of the foramina of Luschka and Magendie).

Communicating hydrocephalus:
- Usually results from a failure of absorption of CSF, due to inflammatory processes, or malignancy in the subarachnoid space.
- Causes include subarachnoid or haemorrhage, meningitis (bacterial, TB and fungal) and carcinomatous meningitis.
- Rarely, a CSF-secreting choroid plexus papilloma can cause a communicating hydrocephalus through overproduction of CSF.

Normal pressure hydrocephalus (*NPH*) (see Chapter 29):
- Usually occurs in the elderly. Patients have normal intracranial pressures.
- It may be either secondary, i.e. a 'low-grade' communicating hydrocephalus due to any of the above causes; or idiopathic, associated with cerebrovascular disease in the elderly.

ASSOCIATIONS/RISK FACTORS
- High incidence in spina bifida patients with open myelomeningocele: 80% will need a shunt.
- A number of genetic syndromic conditions are associated with hydrocephalus: look for other syndromic features.
- Late deterioration in function following head injury can occur due to post-traumatic hydrocephalus.

PATHOLOGY/PATHOGENESIS
- CSF is produced in the cerebral ventricles at a rate of approximately 500–750 mL/day.
- 80% is secreted by the choroid plexus within the ventricles and 20% by transependymal bulk flow of brain interstitial fluid.
- CSF flows through the ventricular system, exiting the fourth ventricle via the foramina of Luschka and Magendie to enter the subarachnoid space.
- CSF absorption occurs via the arachnoid granulations, nerve sheaths, nasal lymphatics and through 'reverse bulk flow' into the brain capillaries.
- CSF production is independent of ICP but the absorption of CSF rises linearly with ICP. Thus, if the flow of CSF through the ventricles is obstructed or if scarring in the subarachnoid space results in the failure of absorption, the CSF production continues resulting in expansion of the ventricles and an increase in intracranial pressure.

HISTORY
- In most situations you will encounter patients who already have a diagnosis of hydrocephalus but where the treatment, either a ventriculoperitoneal (VP) shunt or an endoscopic third ventriculostomy (ETV), has failed and they re-present with recurrent symptoms.

> *Remember: Presentation of these patients is varied—patients or their parents/carers are often right when they suspect VP shunt blockage—ignore them at your peril.*

Infants:
- Abnormal head growth with 'crossing centiles' on growth chart.
- Irritability, vomiting, apnoeic episodes and developmental delay.

Children and younger adults:
- Symptoms of raised intracranial pressure—headaches (typically waking from sleep in early morning, relieved on vomiting and worse on coughing/straining and lying down), nausea and vomiting and visual deterioration.
- Seizures are a relatively uncommon presenting feature but can be confused with 'hydrocephalic attacks'—abrupt collapse with loss of consciousness due to abrupt rise in ICP. Recovery of consciousness can occur, for example due to transient relief of obstruction.

> *Remember: Hydrocephalic attacks are common in patients with obstructive hydrocephalus due to colloid cysts where such events are an ominous sign of impending catastrophic deterioration.*

- More slowly progressive cases may not have headache, only visual failure due to occult optic atrophy and/or disturbance of gait (ataxia) and cognition (e.g. decline in school performance) and urinary incontinence.

Elderly:
- *Triad of symptoms of NPH:* Gait disturbance, dementia and urinary incontinence.

Shunt infection:
- If a shunt has been inserted within the last year there is a risk of it being infected.
- Ask about history of fever, abdominal pain and redness (erythema) along the course of shunt as it passes subcutaneously.

EXAMINATION
Infants:
- Head circumference over 98th centile; tense or full fontanelle; dilated scalp veins.
- Loss of upgaze 'sunsetting' (usually in obstructive hydrocephalus) due to downward pressure on tectum.

Children and younger adults:
- *Signs of raised intracranial pressure:* Decreased level of consciousness/coma, papilloedema and may have loss of upgaze; bilateral VI nerve palsies (false localising sign).
- Gait ataxia.
- Visual acuity, visual fields and fundoscopic findings should be documented in any patient with hydrocephalus or suspected shunt failure.
- Examine for evidence of an existing shunt system, the valve may be felt as a palpable lump under the scalp either on the top of the head behind hairline or a few centimetres above and behind the ear.
- Most shunt valves have a 'reservoir' that can be depressed and felt to refill if shunt is working. The shunt catheter may be palpated as it passes subcutaneously from scalp incision to abdominal incision. Look for any signs of infection of these incisions.

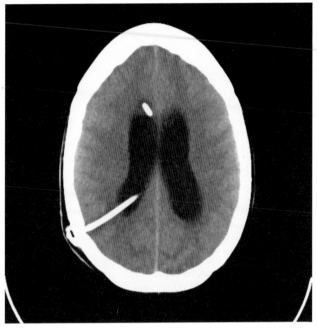

Figure 37.1 CT head scan showing typical enlargement of ventricles. Note the ventricular shunt catheter visible as a radioopaque structure passing into the occipital horn of the right lateral ventricle and part of the proximal catheter of a separate ventricular access device (also known as an Ommaya reservoir) passing into the right frontal horn.

Elderly:
- Usually do *not* have signs of raised ICP. Typically gait ataxia and cognitive impairment only.

INVESTIGATIONS
CT head scan:
- Look for enlargement of ventricles (Evan's ratio (frontal horn width/maximum biparietal diameter) >30%). Pattern of ventricular enlargement helps identify level of obstruction (e.g. in aqueduct stenosis, the IV ventricle is small and the lateral and III ventricles enlarged).
- The VP shunt catheter(s) are visible as a white (radio-opaque) linear structure (Figure 37.1).

Remember: In patients with VP shunts, small ventricles DO NOT exclude shunt failure or raised intracranial pressure; urgent discussion with local neurosurgical team is advised in cases of suspected shunt blockage.

MRI scan:
- Can identify structural abnormalities causing obstructive hydrocephalus (e.g. tumours).

Shunt series:
- Skull AP and lateral, chest and abdominal X-rays.
- To assess continuity of VP shunt system: look for breaks in tubing and/or migration of catheters.

Ultrasound:
- Frequently used in infants with open fontanelle. Useful to monitor ventricular size.

ICP monitoring:
- Used when imaging is equivocal to determine whether ICP is raised.

Lumbar infusion study:
- Lumbar puncture is contraindicated in obstructive hydrocephalus.
- In communicating hydrocephalus, a one off ICP reading with a manometer can assist diagnosis, with drainage of CSF providing temporary symptomatic relief.
- An infusion study is a more sophisticated test measuring dynamic changes in ICP in response to infusion of artificial CSF into the lumbar subarachnoid space; it can be of use in the diagnosis of NPH or can help diagnose shunt blockage.

CSF drainage tests:
- Used in the diagnosis of NPH. Objective testing of gait and cognition before and after large-volume CSF drainage via a lumbar drain over a few days. Improvement in either gait or cognition correlates strongly with shunt responsiveness.

Neuropsychological testing:
- Can be used to monitor children or adults with hydrocephalus. A decline in cognitive performance may indicate shunt malfunction.

MANAGEMENT

Medical Treatment
- Hydrocephalus remains a surgically treated condition.
- Acetazolamide reduces CSF production and can be given as a temporising measure.
- Serial lumbar punctures may temporise hydrocephalus in cases of communicating hydrocephalus.
- If a deteriorating patient with known hydrocephalus has a ventricular access device (a ventricular catheter connected to a blind ending subcutaneous reservoir, usually located in the frontal region and separate from the shunt system) (Figure 37.1), this can be accessed using strict asepsis with a 25G needle to remove CSF in order to temporarily reduce ICP.

Surgical Treatment
Obstructive Hydrocephalus
Removal of cause:
- In some cases, such as tumours or colloid cysts, removal of the obstructing lesion can re-establish CSF flow.

Endoscopic third ventriculostomy (ETV):
- An operation in which a hole is made in the floor of the third ventricle into the sub-arachnoid space below it, allowing the obstruction (in the cerebral aqueduct or posterior fossa) to be 'bypassed'. Successful in around 60% of cases.

Ventriculo-peritoneal (VP) shunt (Figure 37.1):
- A system for draining CSF from the ventricle to the peritoneal cavity, where it is absorbed.
- Three components: a ventricular catheter, which usually lies in the frontal or occipital horn of the lateral ventricle, connected to a valve (usually with an integral reservoir) and a distal catheter, which passes subcutaneously, draining the CSF (when the valve opens) to the peritoneal cavity.
- Other sites used occasionally for distal catheter drainage include the pleural cavity (ventriculo-pleural shunt) and the right atrium, via the internal jugular vein (a ventriculo-atrial (VA) shunt).
- Many different shunt valves are available. Most are differential pressure valves, opening at a fixed pressure. Programmable valves allow adjustment of the valve opening pressure.

Communicating Hydrocephalus and NPH
- These types of hydrocephalus are usually treated with a VP shunt as described above.
- The lumbar subarachnoid space is sometimes used as an alternative to ventricular catheter placement in communicating hydrocephalus, and is known as a lumbo-peritoneal (LP) shunt.

COMPLICATIONS
- Neither VP shunts nor ETV offer permanent cure of the condition; both may block leading to recurrent symptoms of hydrocephalus requiring revision surgery. Untreated hydrocephalus is often fatal.
- Delayed treatment can lead to permanent visual loss or significant cognitive impairment.
- Epilepsy can arise either due to underlying conditions or surgical intervention to treat hydrocephalus.

Shunts
Overdrainage:
- Shunts may drain too much of CSF causing low pressure symptoms such as headaches (typically relieved by lying down) and vomiting; in more severe cases, they can lead to collapse of ventricle that may cause tearing of bridging veins on the brain surface leading to *subdural haematoma* formation.

Infection:
- Rarely occurs more than 1 year after the shunt insertion (*exception*: VA shunts, which can become infected with any bacteraemia).
- Clinical signs include meningism and erythema along the line of distal catheter; confirm diagnosis with CSF culture from shunt reservoir.
- Requires shunt removal in most cases.
- Infected VA shunts can lead to renal failure due to shunt nephritis and pulmonary hypertension due to microemboli.

Blockage:
- Can occur at any time after shunt insertion, sometimes many decades later.
- Patients present with recurrent symptoms and signs of hydrocephalus.

Migration, disconnection, breakage of shunt catheters:
- Can be a cause of shunt failure. Look for evidence of loss of continuity of tubing on shunt series.

ETV
Blockage:
- Can still occur following ETV, often many years later and can be associated with fatality if not recognised. Clinical features of recurrent hydrocephalus.

PROGNOSIS
Untreated:
- Fatal in approximately 80% of cases. Sixty per cent of survivors left with significant learning disability.
- Twenty per cent of survivors are blind.

Treated:
- Risk of mortality from shunt-related problems is 1–3% per year.
- With treatment, patients can expect to undergo regular shunt revisions.
- Infants have a 50% shunt failure rate within 1 year. Older children and adults on average undergo two shunt revisions every 10 years.
- Cognitive outcome is dictated by the presence of associated underlying conditions, although repeated episodes of raised ICP due to shunt complications or the development of an associated seizure disorder can have an adverse effect on cognition.
- Raised ICP due to hydrocephalus can lead to progressive optic atrophy with visual failure.

DIFFERENTIAL DIAGNOSIS (TABLE 37.1)

Table 37.1 Differential diagnoses of ventricular enlargement and of VP shunt failure.

Ventricular enlargement	
External hydrocephalus	• Macrocephaly and enlarged subarachnoid spaces with mild ventriculomegaly in the first year of life • Typically asymptomatic with normal development, benign and self-limiting • Differentiate from communicating hydrocephalus and subdural effusions • Serial lumbar punctures occasionally required to prevent cosmetically unacceptable head growth • Some cases associated with neonatal lupus
Ex vacuo ventricular dilatation	• Usually seen in the elderly or in association with genetic disorders that cause cerebral atrophy • As the cranial cavity is of fixed dimensions, when the brain parenchymal volume decreases, the ventricles enlarge to occupy the space vacated by the brain • There is no disturbance of CSF circulation • Differentiate from NPH on CT/MR imaging and with lumbar infusion study
Arrested/compensated hydrocephalus	• Finding of ventriculomegaly in an asymptomatic adult patient • Macrocephaly is usually present, due to compensation of hydrocephalus in early life • No symptoms or signs of raised ICP present • Small risk of late decompensation, often with NPH features or occult visual failure
Hydranencephaly	• Congenital absence of cerebrum with normal meninges and cranial vault • May have progressive macrocephaly • Cranial cavity is filled with CSF • Differentiate from severe congenital hydrocephalus with MRI and absence of cortical activity on EEG • Prognosis is poor—usually death in infancy

VP shunt failure

- The presentation of patients with VP shunt blockage is notoriously variable
- In children, systemic infection may mimic the early symptoms of raised ICP
- Patients with spina bifida are prone to UTIs which should be considered in the differential diagnosis
- Drug side effects and seizures may also mimic symptoms of shunt malfunction

Remember: The consequences of missing shunt failure are severe, so this diagnosis should be actively excluded.

Appendices

1   Management of status epilepticus (SE)*

- *SE*: Continuous seizures lasting >30 min or multiple seizures without full recovery of consciousness in between seizures.
- SE can occur in all forms of seizures (e.g. partial or complex partial status); the commonest type, however, presenting as an emergency is the convulsive primary or secondary generalised tonic–clonic SE.
- *Commonest scenario*: A patient with a known seizure disorder and subtherapeutic antiepileptic drug (AED) levels due to non-compliance or other factors. Other causes include cerebrovascular accidents in elderly, CNS infection, first presentation of epilepsy, electrolyte disturbances, for example hyponatraemia or hypoglycaemia or hypocalcaemia, alcohol withdrawal, head injury and CNS tumours.
- Treat any seizure lasting >10 min aggressively. Adequate management of SE also includes trying to prevent its future recurrence; therefore, address non-compliance with respect to AED intake if applicable.
- Management includes the following:
  - Airway and breathing (maintain the airway using oral/nasal adjuncts and intubation if necessary; administer oxygen using bag valve mask).
  - Obtain IV access and bloods for investigations (as above and including anticonvulsant levels and toxicology screen if appropriate and fingerstick glucose value). Maintain blood pressure well using intravenous fluids if necessary.
  - In unknown patients or in cases of malnourished or alcoholic patients, administer intravenous thiamine followed by a glucose bolus (unless glucose known to be normal), for example IV glucose 50 mL of 50%.
  - In ongoing seizures, administer lorazepam intravenously (2–4 mg average adult dose at a rate of <2 mg/min) or intravenous diazepam (5–10 mg average adult dose at a rate of 5 mg/min). Doses can be repeated. A major side effect is respiratory depression, which may necessitate intubation and therefore resuscitation facility should be available at all times.
  - Load with phenytoin 15 mg/kg IV at a rate of ≤50 mg/min with ECG and BP monitoring due to risk of *hypotension and arrhythmias*. Start maintenance therapy with phenytoin PO thereafter for the emergent period or longer.
  - With continuing seizures, other agents such as phenobarbital can be used in an intensive care setting.
  - Continuing seizures despite above need specialist input with induction of general anaesthesia and continuous EEG monitoring with maintenance of burst suppression in ITU.
  - Remember to inform and involve the anaesthetists or intensive care physicians as soon as possible.

*See Chapter 17.

2 Glasgow Coma Scale (GCS)

Developed in 1974 by Jennett and Teasdale, this scoring system is now used worldwide in the assessment of head injuries, although a 15-point scale (Table A1) has now largely replaced the original 14-point scale (which omitted the 'abnormal flexion' category).

> *Remember: The individual elements of the score as well as the sum are important and both should be expressed, for example GCS 11 (E3, V2, M6).*

The severity of the head injury can be grouped according to the GCS:
- *Mild*: GCS $\geq$13.
- *Moderate*: GCS 9–12.
- *Severe*: GCS $\leq$8.

The score is used in both the initial assessment of head-injured patients and as the basis for neurological observations to detect any secondary deterioration.

Table A1 The Glasgow Coma Scale

Score	Component	Notes
Motor (M)		Denotes *best* response from either upper limb
6	Obeys commands	For example 'wiggle your fingers'. Do *not* use 'squeeze my hand' as this may elicit a grasp reflex response. Can use 'stick out tongue'; 'blink twice' if suspected/proven high cervical cord injury. Always test before inflicting painful stimuli!
5	Localises pain	Usually supraorbital pressure (to supraorbital nerve in supraorbital groove), positive if hand moves above chin
4	Flexion/withdrawal to pain	Finger nailbed compression– withdraws upper limb *or* flexion of elbow, supination of forearm and flexion of wrist when supraorbital pressure applied
3	Abnormal flexion to pain (decorticate posturing)	Adduction of arm, internal rotation of shoulder, elbow flexion, pronation of forearm, flexion of wrist and extension of lower extremities to supraorbital pressure
2	Extension to pain (decerebrate posturing)	Adduction of arm, internal rotation of shoulder, elbow extension, pronation of forearm, wrist

		extension, flexion of fingers and extension of lower extremities to supraorbital pressure	
1	None	No response to pain	
Verbal (V) (older children and adults)		Can add modifier '(d)' for dysphasic if focal speech output disturbance in otherwise alert patient	Paediatric verbal score (*young children (<5 years)*)
5	Orientated	To time, place and person. Responds coherently to questions in sentences	Alert, babbles, coos, words or sentences to usual ability
4	Sentences, confused	Disorientated, confused speech, *but sentences*	Less than usual ability and/or spontaneous irritable cry
3	Occasional/inappropriate words	No conversational speech, random or exclamatory utterances	Cries inappropriately
2	Incomprehensible sounds (moans/groans)	Vocalised moaning but no words	Occasionally whimpers and/or moans
1	None	Can add modifier '(t)' for intubated patient, i.e. V1t	None

Eye opening (E)

4	Spontaneous	
3	To speech	Needs prompting with verbal command to open eyes, i.e. 'pathological drowsiness'. *Note*: Awaking an 'appropriately' (e.g. at night) sleeping individual who remains fully alert once roused should score 4 not 3
2	To pain	Eyes open in response to nailbed pressure or sternal rub (supraorbital pressure not recommended as may cause 'protective' eye closure in response to threat)
1	None	Can use modifier 'c' for closed where eyes cannot open due to periorbital swelling, i.e. E1c

3   Primary neuroepithelial tumours of the central nervous system

	Typical location	Clinical and epidemiological features	Radiology	Pathology	Treatment
Astrocytic tumours					
Pilocytic astrocytoma (WHO Grade I)	Optic pathway (especially neurofibromatosis type 1); cerebral hemisphere; posterior fossa; spinal cord	Most common paediatric posterior fossa tumour; optic nerve lesions may present as painless proptosis. Chiasm lesions may cause field loss +/− pituitary/hypothalamic dysfunction (e.g. precocious puberty)	Well circumscribed, enhancing, frequently have cystic component with 'mural nodule'	Histology: Rosenthal fibres characteristic; vascular proliferation, multinucleated giant cells; occasional mitoses and necrosis may be seen but do not influence survival	Maximal surgical resection achievable without causing deficit is treatment of choice; Optic pathway or incompletely resected lesions: chemotherapy for younger children, radiotherapy if older
Astrocytoma (WHO Grade II)	Throughout CNS, including spinal cord	Children and young adults. Often present with seizures	Hypodense on CT, rarely enhance; hypointense on T1WI MRI	Histological subtypes: fibrillary, gemistocytic (poorest prognosis) and protoplasmic. Dedifferentiation to more malignant tumour occurs	Biopsy. Resection if feasible and clinical or radiological progression. Adjuvant radiotherapy increases progression-free survival, but not overall survival compared to salvage radiotherapy. Salvage chemotherapy
Anaplastic astrocytoma (AA) (WHO Grade III) and **glioblastoma multiforme (GBM) (WHO Grade IV)**	Throughout CNS, including spinal cord. When crosses corpus callosum, it is	AA middle-aged adults (mean 45 years). GBM older age (mean 55 years). **GBM** *most common (50%) parenchymal primary brain tumour.* 10% arise from dedifferentiation of	Irregular, ring-enhancing lesions	High-grade gliomas. *Necrosis with pseudo-palisading of tumour cells and prominent vascular proliferation* differentiate GBM from anaplastic astrocytoma	Maximal surgical resection with adjuvant radiotherapy and chemotherapy (temozolamide). Prognosis influenced by age, performance status,

	known as a 'butterfly glioma'	lower grade astrocytomas. Associations: Li Fraumeni and Turcot syndromes. Fast growing. Metastases throughout CNS but rarely outside CNS			presentation with seizures and treatment. Mean survival 9–12 months
Diffuse pontine glioma	Pons, extending into adjacent brainstem	Malignant tumour. Presentation with combination of cranial nerve palsies and long tract signs, hydrocephalus is a late feature	Diffuse tumour-expanding pons, may encase basilar artery and patchy enhancement may be seen	Anaplastic astrocytoma or GBM histologically	Usually radiological diagnosis; biopsy not necessary unless atypical imaging. Treated with radiotherapy and chemotherapy. Very poor prognosis, death usually within 6–12 months
Subependymal giant cell astrocytoma (SEGA) (WHO Grade I)	Foramen of Monro	Seen in tuberous sclerosis. Presentation: acute obstructive hydrocephalus and seizures	Mass lesion at foramen of Monro with other features of tuberous sclerosis (see Chapter 17)	Genetic defect in either hamartin or tuberin genes– which form tumour suppressor complex of mTOR pathway	Surgical resection or mTOR inhibitors such as everolimus
Tectal glioma	Tectal plate (dorsal midbrain)	A cause of aqueduct stenosis, leading to obstructive hydrocephalus	Tectal plate mass causing obstructive hydrocephalus	Usually low-grade gliomas or hamartomas. Not usually biopsied unless radiological progression occurs	Treat associated hydrocephalus (see Chapter 37). Radiological surveillance and biopsy if progresses
Pleomorphic xanthoastrocytoma (PXA) (WHO Grade I)	Superficial cortex	Rare. Young adults. Commonly present with seizures	Typically superficial, cystic, with	A mixed glioneuronal tumour. Pleomorphic cells	Surgical resection

(Continued)

(Continued)

	Typical location	Clinical and epidemiological features	Radiology	Pathology	Treatment
			enhancing mural nodule	with *lipidisation*. Associated with cortical dysplasia	
Oligodendroglial tumours					
Oligodendroglioma (WHO Grade II or III (anaplastic)	Ninety per cent supratentorial, mainly frontal lobes	Seizures are a common presentation. Mean age 35 years	Mass lesion often with calcification	Tumour cells have 'fried egg' cytoplasm; 'chicken wire' vasculature. Genetic deletions of 1p, 19q associated with better prognosis	Can consider watchful waiting for asymptomatic Grade II tumours. Surgical resection with adjuvant chemotherapy (PCV (procarbazine, CCNU, Vincristine) or temozolamide); +/- radiotherapy for anaplastic tumours
Ependymal tumours					
Subependymoma (WHO Grade I)	IV ventricle or anterior lateral ventricle	Very slow growing, may cause hydrocephalus/mass effect symptoms	Well circumscribed solid mass lesions	Hypocellular tumour with clusters of tumour cells in fibrillar matrix	Surgical resection of symptomatic lesions
Ependymoma (WHO Grade II and III (anaplastic))	IV ventricle, cerebello-pontine angle, cerebral hemispheres and spinal cord	Seventy per cent occur in children; present with hydrocephalus or mass effect symptoms. Spinal cord common location in adults	Solid, variable enhancement	Perivascular pseudo-rosettes. Express GFAP and S100 protein	Radical surgical resection with adjuvant radiotherapy or proton beam therapy; chemotherapy in infants or relapse

Myxopapillary ependymoma	Filum terminale of spinal cord	Adults, present with back pain and symptoms of conus/cauda equina compression	Solid mass lesion in filum terminale	Low-grade tumour. Papillary architecture and myxoid stromal core	Surgical resection curative

Embryonal tumours

Cerebral and spinal primitive neuroectodermal tumour (PNET)	Cerebral hemispheres, brainstem and spinal cord	Children; less common than medulloblastoma	Solid, enhancing mass lesion	Neural crest tumour (as Ewing's sarcoma); Homer–Wright rosettes; frequent mitoses	Surgical resection, chemotherapy +/– radiotherapy (if over 3 years of age)
Medulloblastoma	Roof of IV ventricle	Children; presentation with symptoms of hydrocephalus; spinal 'drop' metastases common. Associated with Gorlin and Turcot syndromes	Solid, midline, enhancing posterior fossa mass	As for PNET	Surgical resection, chemotherapy +/– radiotherapy (over 3 years of age), up to 80% 5-year survival
Atypical teratoid rhabdoid tumour (ATRT)	Posterior fossa (60%)	Rare. Usually children <3 years of age; highly malignant; spinal 'drop' metastases common	Large enhancing mass with calcification, necrosis and haemorrhage often seen	Rhabdoid cells. Absent INI1 antibody staining (distinguishes from PNET)	Surgical resection, chemotherapy +/– radiotherapy

(Continued)

(Continued)

	Typical location	Clinical and epidemiological features	Radiology	Pathology	Treatment
Retinoblastoma	Retina	Leukocoria (absent red reflex (loss of 'red eye' on photographs))	Retinal mass lesion on MRI or orbital ultrasound	As for PNET	Chemotherapy +/− surgical enucleation/radiotherapy
Pineal tumours					
Pineocytoma (WHO Grade II)	Pineal gland	Young adults. Slow growing tumour. Causes obstructive hydrocephalus due to cerebral aqueduct compression	Pineal mass lesion	Tumour cells form 'pineocytomatous rosettes'	Treat associated hydrocephalus; surgical resection if symptomatic mass effect
Pineoblastoma (WHO Grade IV)	Pineal gland	Presentation with obstructive hydrocephalus	Pineal mass lesion	Histologically, has features of PNET.	Surgical resection, chemotherapy +/− radiotherapy
Miscellaneous rare tumours					
Ganglioglioma (WHO Grade I)	Cerebral hemispheres, especially temporal lobe	Children and young adults; slow growing, often present with seizures	Often calcified; partly cystic	Mixture of neuronal (ganglion cells) and glial (astrocytes) tumour cells	Surgical excision if possible

Dysembryoplastic neuroepithelial tumour (DNET) (WHO Grade I)	Cortical lesions typically temporal or frontal lobes	Children and young adults; slow growing, often present with seizures	MRI: well defined, hypointense on T1WI and hyperintense on T2 WI. Hypodense on CT with remodelling of overlying calvaria	Glioneuronal elements; may be associated with cortical dysplasia	Surgical resection if possible to control seizures
Central neurocytoma (WHO Grade II)	Lateral ventricles	Young adults	Enhancing intraventricular mass lesion	Similar to oligodendroglioma, differentiated on immunostaining (synaptophysin positive)	Complete surgical resection is curative
Choroid plexus papilloma (WHO grade I)	Ventricles	Infants and young children, usually supratentorial. When occur in adults, infratentorial location most common. May present with hydrocephalus due to CSF overproduction (see Chapter 37)	Intraventricular, lobulated, enhancing mass, little parenchymal oedema	Papillary architecture covered with single layer of columnar epithelial cells, cellular pleomorphism but no mitoses	Surgical excision is curative
Choroid plexus carcinoma (WHO Grade IV)	Ventricles	Infants and young children. Associated with Li Fraumeni syndrome.	Similar to papilloma but marked surrounding oedema and tumour extension into surrounding parenchyma	Rapid growing malignant tumour; frequent mitoses, necrosis	Surgical excision, adjuvant chemotherapy and radiotherapy

(Continued)

(*Continued*)

	Typical location	Clinical and epidemiological features	Radiology	Pathology	Treatment
Haemangioblastoma	Cerebellum	Most common primary posterior fossa tumour in adults. Associated with **Von Hippel Lindau disease** (multiple haemangioblastomas; renal cell carcinoma and retinal angiomatosis; renal and pancreatic cysts; polycythemia; phaeochromocytoma)	Solid or cystic with enhancing mural nodule. Radiological screening for other features of VHL	Highly vascular tumours composed of stromal tumour cells of unknown origin	Surgical resection if possible

Note: Tumours highlighted in bold are important for exams.

4 Other tumours affecting the central nervous system

	Typical location	Clinical and epidemiological features	Radiology	Pathology	Treatment
Metastases	Throughout CNS. Frequently multiple. May infiltrate leptomeninges (carcinomatous meningitis) causing multiple cranial nerve palsies	**Most common intracranial tumour**. Incidence increasing. **Lung, breast, renal, GI** and **melanoma** most common primary sites. Presenting symptom in 15% with no previous history of malignancy. Malignant cells on LP in carcinomatous meningitis	Often well circumscribed, enhancing lesions, typically located at grey–white matter junction. May be 'ring enhancing'. Often multiple. MRI more sensitive for multiple lesions. Get CT chest, abdomen and pelvis to look for primary/other metastases	Cytokeratin positive immunostaining for carcinomas	Biopsy to confirm diagnosis of solitary lesion +/– surgical resection or Stereotactic Radiosurgery; radiotherapy for widespread metastases or leptomeningeal spread. Chemotherapy for some primary types
Cerebral lymphoma	Frontal lobe or periventricular location most common for primary (usually B-cell) CNS lymphoma. Secondary (usually T-cell) CNS lymphomas typically diffuse leptomeningeal infiltration (positive CSF cytology)	Associated with Immunosuppression (AIDS; posttransplant) and collagen vascular disease (SLE; Sjogren's; rheumatoid arthritis). Presentation as for other CNS tumours, may also present with dementia without focal signs	On CT, 60% are hyperdense to brain. Homogenous enhancing lesions or multifocal ring-enhancing lesions on CT/MRI. No pathognomic features	Perivascular cuffing of lymphoma cells; immunostaining to differentiate cell type: B-cell CD20 positive; T-cell CD45 positive	Systemic evaluation for lymphoma (clinical exam + CT chest, abdomen and pelvis; bone marrow biopsy; testicular ultrasound). Rapid initial response to steroids (tumour may transiently disappear); surgical resection does not affect prognosis (do biopsy only); treat with whole brain radiotherapy +/– chemotherapy

(Continued)

(Continued)

	Typical location	Clinical and epidemiological features	Radiology	Pathology	Treatment
Meningioma	Commonest locations falx, cerebral convexity and sphenoid wing. Can arise in spinal canal	**Most common primary intracranial tumour.** Slow growing, often asymptomatic (3% of autopsies in >60 years old). Middle age and older adults; rare in children	Homogenous, enhancing mass arising from inner surface of skull vault; overlying hyperostosis of skull may be seen; may be calcified; 'streak' of adjacent dural enhancement may be seen—a 'dural tail'	Arise from arachnoid cap cells. 'Psammoma bodies' seen on histology. 'Atypical' and 'malignant' meningiomas (<5% of all) show increased mitotic activity	Surgical resection or Stereotactic radiosurgery. Small, asymptomatic meningiomas may be monitored with surveillance imaging
Schwannoma	Spinal nerve roots ('dumbell' tumours extending either side of neural foramen) or cranial nerves. Usually on sensory roots. Most common is VIII cranial nerve, 'acoustic neuroma' (a misnomer) which arises on vestibular division of the nerve (i.e. it is a vestibular schwannoma)	Acoustic neuroma presents in middle age with unilateral sensorineural deafness and balance difficulties; larger lesions cause headaches and facial weakness and numbness from V and VII nerve compression. Bilateral acoustic neuromas diagnostic of neurofibromatosis type 2 (inactivation of 'schwannomin' gene;	Intradural, extramedullary, enhancing lesions best seen on MRI. Acoustic neuromas expand the internal auditory meatus on CT	Encapsulated, benign tumours, histologically composed of Antoni A (compact, spindle-shaped and bipolar cells) and Antoni B (loose reticulated cells within matrix) fibres. S-100 positive on immunostaining	Small lesions with minimal symptoms may be observed. Stereotactic Radiosurgery for small tumours. Surgical resection (retrosigmoid approach for hearing preservation; translabyrinthine approach, sacrifices hearing but possible improved VII preservation) for larger tumours with stereotactic radiosurgery for any residuum.

	chromosome 22). Spinal schwannomas present with progressive symptoms and signs of spinal cord compression			Peripheral schwannomas may be excised with preservation of other nerve fascicles
Neurofibroma	Skin: 'dermal neurofibromas'. Plexiform neurofibromas arise in skin or internal nerve bundles; they are often very large and disfiguring, involve multiple tissue layers and are associated with overlying cutaneous overgrowth. Can arise on spinal nerve roots resulting in cord compression	Multiple lesions, usually seen in type 1 neurofibromatosis. Plexiform neurofibromas: large multilobulated masses	Not encapsulated, arise from peripheral nerve schwann cells. Encase or invade other fascicles of nerve. Microscopy shows schwann cell, axonal and fibroblast elements. Ten per cent of plexiform lesions undergo malignant transformation to malignant peripheral nerve sheath tumour	In NF1 surgery for cosmesis, neural compression or if rapidly enlarging. Complete excision usually involves nerve root sacrifice which may worsen neurological deficit
Pituitary tumours				
Pituitary adenoma (functional (secrete pituitary hormones); or non-functional)	Usually arise in middle age; some associated with multiple endocrine neoplasia (MEN). *Non-functioning adenomas* present with symptoms of mass effect, for example optic chiasm compression (bitemporal haemianopia); hypopituitarism; cavernous sinus	Pituitary fossa (sellar), with suprasellar extension causing compression of optic chiasm. MRI preferred. Tumour usually solid, intrasellar mass, may have suprasellar extension with chiasm compression. Haemorrhage present in pituitary apoplexy. Pituitary fossa may be expanded on skull X-ray	Termed microadenoma if <1 cm in diameter. *Microscopy:* Chromophobe adenoma commonly 'non-secretory' tumour; acidophil adenoma usually growth hormone secreting or prolactinoma; basophil adenoma usually ACTH secreting (Cushing's	Emergency surgery for apoplexy with visual loss; surgery for non-functioning tumours or local mass effect (e.g. visual field loss) and tissue diagnosis. Surgery usually via transnasal, transsphenoidal route. Some secretory tumours can be managed medically

(Continued)

(Continued)

	Typical location	Clinical and epidemiological features	Radiology	Pathology	Treatment
		compression (pressure on III, IV and VI causing diplopia, ptosis(II); V (first and second divisions) causing facial pain). *Functional adenomas:* Prolactin secreting—amenorrhoea—galactorrhoea syndrome (infertility; impotence in males); ACTH secreting—Cushing's disease; growth hormone secreting—acromegaly (rarely gigantism in children); thyrotrophin (TSH) secreting (rare)—thyrotoxicosis		disease). Immunostaining can define secretory products	(e.g. **Prolactinoma: bromocriptine, cabergoline. Growth hormone secreting tumour: octreotide**).
Craniopharyngioma	Suprasellar region, third ventricle	More common in children, often present with hypopituitarism, visual field loss (bitemporal haemianopia) or with	Part solid and cystic or multicystic tumours in suprasellar region; often calcified on CT	Cysts lined with stratified squamous epithelium and contain cholesterol crystals	Surgical resection or debulking +/− CSF shunt for associated hydrocephalus. Radiotherapy or intracyst instillation of bleomycin is

	Location	Clinical features	Imaging	Pathology / markers	Treatment
		headaches due to associated hydrocephalus			also used. Treatment of associated hypopituitarism and diabetes insipidus often required
Rathke's cleft cyst	Sellar or suprasellar region	Usually asymptomatic, may cause visual field disturbance or hypopituitarism/diabetes insipidus	Hypodense cystic lesions on CT, lining may enhance	Arise from Rathke's pouch remnant in pars intermedia of pituitary gland; cyst of single-layer cuboidal epithelium contains 'motor oil' fluid	If symptomatic, treat with transsphenoidal drainage and biopsy only
Germ cell tumours (GCT) [(Germinoma; non-germinomatous germ cell tumours (embryonal carcinoma, yolk sac a.k.a endodermal sinus tumour, choriocarcinoma); teratoma (mature or immature)]	Occur in the midline: pineal gland and suprasellar region	Often present with hydrocephalus due to aqueduct obstruction. In boys only, GCTs (choriocarcinoma or germinoma) may present with precocious puberty due to βHCG secretion. Tumours (except mature teratoma) are malignant and can disseminate throughout CNS and metastases can present with signs of spinal cord compression	Pineal or suprasellar mass lesion; simultaneous bifocal lesions usually germinoma	GCTs often secrete tumour markers found in serum and CSF: **βHCG (choriocarcinoma (all) and 10% of germinomas); alpha fetoprotein (AFP) (endodermal sinus tumour).** If positive, can be used to monitor treatment. Tumours may contain mixed cell populations. Mature teratomas are encapsulated and contain tissue derived from all three germ layers and often contain identifiable tissues	Associated obstructive hydrocephalus treated with endoscopic third ventriculostomy with biopsy if serum and CSF tumour markers are negative. Many GCTs are very chemo- and radiosensitive; surgical resection is reserved for teratomas and tumours resistant to adjuvant therapy

(Continued)

(Continued)

	Typical location	Clinical and epidemiological features	Radiology	Pathology	Treatment
				such as teeth and hair; the tissues within them may undergo malignant transformation	
Epidermoid and dermoid tumours	Scalp and skull vault. Epidermoid: Cerebello-pontine angle, suprasellar. Dermoid: midline	Present with symptoms of local mass effect. Cyst rupture causes aseptic (Mollaret's) meningitis. Repeated bacterial meningitis seen in spinal dermoid cysts with associated dermal sinus tract	Epidermoid cysts are hypodense on CT and on MRI are similar to CSF (hypointense on T1 and hyperintense on T2-weighted imaging), but on diffusion weighted MR imaging have restricted diffusion, differentiating them from arachnoid cysts. Dermoid cysts are hyperintense (like fat) on T1-weighted imaging due to the presence of cholesterol and have heterogeneous appearance on T2-	Embryologically, both of ectodermal origin. They are hamartomas, so growth is linear (not exponential). Epidermoid cysts are lined by stratified squamous epithelium and contain keratin and cholesterol (hence also known as cholesteatoma). Dermoid cysts lined by dermis, containing hair follicles, apocrine and sebaceous glands. Contain cellular debris and gland secretions, may also contain hair and teeth	Surgical resection with steroid cover to reduce risk of chemical meningitis and postoperative hydrocephalus. Tumours are *not* radiosensitive

		weighted imaging. Ruptured cysts show fat droplets in subarachnoid cisterns		
Glomus jugulare tumours	Pulsatile mass visible behind eardrum. Cerebello-pontine angle mass	Unilateral hearing loss (conductive or sensorineural) and pulsatile tinnitus and lower cranial nerve palsies. Tumours may secrete catecholamines with similar symptoms to phaeochromocytoma. Rare, but most common middle ear neoplasm. F:M = 6:1	CT to assess bony destruction of middle ear and petrous temporal bone; MRI to evaluate CP angle component and assess jugular bulb patency	May secrete catecholamines, serotonin and histamines. Urine may be positive for VMA. Histologically, same as carotid body tumours. Encapsulated and highly vascular	Preoperative embolisation to devascularise tumour. Surgical resection or stereotactic radiosurgery. Alpha and beta blockade required pre-operatively for catecholamine secreting tumours

Note: Tumours highlighted in bold are important for exams.

Index

acetazolamide, 54
acoustic neuroma, 15, 21, 39, 40, 177
acute subdural haematoma (ASDH), 135, 136, 138, 143. *See also* head injury
  aetiology, 135
  CT scan, 136
  history, 135
  mortality rates, 138
AED. *See* antiepileptic drug (AED)
ALS. *See* amyotrophic lateral sclerosis (ALS)
Alzheimer's disease (AD), 118–21
  aetiology, 118
  associations/risk factors, 118
  complications, 120
  differential diagnoses, 120–1
  epidemiology, 118
  examination, 119
  history, 118–19
  investigations, 119
  management, 119–20
  pathology/pathogenesis, 118
  prognosis, 120
amaurosis fugax, 37, 53, 55
amitriptyline, 52
  for chronic tension-type headaches, 52
  to reduce neuropathy-related discomfort, 102
amyotrophic lateral sclerosis (ALS), 22, 23, 42, 43, 108
aneurysm, 23–5, 71, 72
  intracranial, 68
  mycotic, 65
  treatment of, 72, 73
antiepileptic drug (AED), 77, 78, 128, 165
antiplatelet agents, 56, 62
artery
  angiography, 25, 55, 67, 153
  basilar, 5, 6, 170
  carotid, 6, 25, 53, 55, 59, 60
    internal, 5
  cerebral, 54, 60, 65, 68, 70, 72, 73, 125
    anterior, 5, 6
    middle, 5, 6
    posterior, 5, 6, 8
  anterior inferior cerebellar, 5
  posterior inferior cerebellar, 5
  cortical, 135
  femoral, 25
  meningeal, 141
  occlusion, 8, 37, 60, 72
  ophthalmic, 37, 55
  retinal, 55
  spinal, 5, 144
  temporal, 53, 54
  vertebral, 5, 25, 68, 146
ASDH, 135. *See* acute subdural haematoma (ASDH)
aspirin, 52, 56, 61

  for antiplatelet agents, 56
  for headache, 52
  in intracerebral haemorrhage, 67
  for thromboembolic stroke, 61, 62
atorvastatin, 62
attention deficit hyperactivity disorder (ADHD), 131
autonomic dysreflexia, 146

Becker muscular dystrophy, 117
beta-blockers, 56, 87, 111
blackouts, 34–5
  after the attack, 35
  during the attack, 35
  carotid sinus massage, 35
  clinical conditions, 34
  differential diagnoses
    basic investigations, 35
    basic management, 35
  prior to attack, 34
  selected questions to ask/facts to establish, 34
  syncope *vs.* seizures, 34
blood alcohol level, 132
botulism, 113
brainstem, 4–5
  auditory evoked potentials, 21
  death, 127 (*See also* coma)
    criteria for diagnosis, 129
  vertebrobasilar system, 6

caffeine intake, 27
carbamazepine, 54, 77, 78, 82
carcinomatous meningitis, 26, 155, 176. *See also* meningitis
carotid endarterectomy, 63
carpal tunnel syndrome (CTS), 7, 100, 104
cauda equina syndrome (CES), 41, 44, 97, 98, 99
central nervous system
  clinical syndromes related to pathology, 8
  infections, 91, 93–6 (*See also* cerebral abscess; meningitis)
  neoplasia, 151–4
  primary neuroepithelial tumours (*See* tumours)
cerebellum, 5, 6, 46, 65, 81, 126
cerebral abscess, 93–6
  aetiology, 94
  complications, 96
  defined, 94
  differential diagnoses, 96
  examination, 94
  history, 94
  investigations, 94–5
    T1- and T2-weighted images, 95
  management, 95–6
  pathology/pathogenesis, 94
  prognosis, 96

cerebral herniation, 125–6
cerebral oedema, 122
cerebral spinal fluid (CSF)
    analysis, 25–7, 32, 68, 70, 82, 101, 124
    different clinical conditions, and finding, 26
    drainage tests, 158
    nasal CSF leaks, 133
    otorrhoea, 133
    shunt infections, 93
cerebral vasospasm, treatment and preventions, 72–3
cervical cord injury, 134
cervical spine fractures, 148
chorea, 89
    aetiology, 89
    defined, 89
chronic inflammatory demyelinating
    polyneuropathy (CIDP), 42, 101, 103
chronic subdural haematomas (CSDH), 135,
    136, 138
clopidogrel, 56, 62, 67
cluster headache, 53
    epidemiology, 53
    history, 53
    investigations, 53
    management, 53
CNS neoplasia, 151–4
    complications, 153
    differential diagnoses, 153–4
    examination, 151
    history, 151
    investigations, 151–3
        CT scans, 153
    management, 153
    pathology, 151
    prognosis, 153
coma, 127–9, 134
    aetiology, 127
    associations/risk factors, 127
    complications, 128–9
    defined, 127
    differential diagnoses, 129
    examination, 127
    history, 127
    investigations, 128
    management, 128
    pathology/pathogenesis, 127
    prognosis, 129
contusions
    aetiology, 135
    associations/ risk factors, 135
    clinical conditions, 139
    complications, 138
    CT scan, 136–8, 140
    defined, 135
    differential diagnosis, 143
    epidemiology, 135
    examination, 136–7
    history, 135
    investigations, 137–8
    management, 138
    pathology/pathogenesis, 135
    prognosis, 138
cortical anatomy, 4

cranial nerves (CN), 4–5
cytotoxic oedema, 123

Dabigatran, 56
deep venous thrombosis (DVT), 62, 63, 103,
    146, 147
Dementia pugilistica, 134
dementia syndromes, 118–21
    differential diagnoses, 120–1
dermatomes
    anterior and posterior aspects of body, 19
    cotton wool/fingertip, 19
dexamethasone, 42, 92, 122, 123, 125, 153
diazepam
    for seizures, 165
    side effect, 165
diffuse axonal injury (DAI), 130
diplopia, 11, 14, 60, 78, 112, 133, 178
dipyridamole
    for thromboembolic stroke, 62
    for transient ischaemic attacks (TIAs), 56
disc herniation, 97. See also radiculopathy
dizziness, 39
    clinical conditions, 39–40
    differential diagnoses, 39
    selected questions to ask/facts to
        establish, 39
double vision. See diplopia
Duchenne muscular dystrophy, 117
dysdiadochokinesis, 20
dystonia, 88, 90
    aetiology, 90
    defined, 90
    investigation, 90
    management, 90

encephalitis, 31, 93
endoscopic third ventriculostomy (ETV), 156,
    158, 159
epilepsy, 73, 75
    aetiology, 75
    associations/risk factors, 76
    characteristics, 75
    classification, 75
    complications, 78
    defined, 75
    epidemiology, 75
    examination, 76–7
    history, 76
    investigations, 77
    management, 77–9 (See also status
        epilepticus (SE))
        newer AEDs, 78
        phenytoin as effective drug, 77
    partial seizures, 75–6
    pathology/pathogenesis, 76
    primary generalised seizures, 75
    prognosis, 78
        mortality rates, 78
    temporal lobe epilepsy, 119
extradural haematoma
    acute, large left-sided, 142
    aetiology, 141
    associations/risk factors, 141

complications, 143
defined, 141
differential diagnoses, 143
epidemiology, 141
examination, 141–2
history, 141
investigation, 142
   CT scan, 142
management, 143
pathology/pathogenesis, 141
prognosis, 143
spinal, 27, 42, 99

folic acid, 78
frontotemporal dementia, 120

gabapentin, 54, 89
gait assessment/disturbance, 8, 16, 20, 158
aetiology, 46
broad-based gait, 47
clinical conditions, 46–7
differential diagnoses, 46–7
extrapyramidal disorder, 47
foot drop, 47
localisation, 46
selected questions to ask/facts to
   establish, 46
spastic hemiparesis/paraparesis, 46–7
waddling gait, 47
GBS. See Guillain-Barré syndrome (GBS)
giant cell arteritis (GCA), 31, 53–4
Glasgow coma scale (GCS), 166–7
glossopharyngeal nerves, 5
Guillain–Barré syndrome (GBS), 25, 41, 42,
   101–3
aetiology, 102
defined, 102
epidemiology, 102
examination, 102
history, 102
investigations, 102
management, 103
pathology/pathogenesis, 102

Hangman's fracture, 148
HD. See Huntington's disease (HD)
headache
acute/chronic, 31
as complications, 27
   history of, 31
conditions causing
   giant cell arteritis, 53
   idiopathic intracranial hypertension, 53
   trigeminal neuralgia, 54
defined, 51
differential diagnoses
   basic investigations, 32–3
   basic management, 33
duration of, 31
episodic, 31
Kernig's sign, 32
lumbar puncture (LP), 32
neurology clinics, 31
pain in face, 32

past medical history, 32
points to consider, 32
selected questions to ask/facts to
   establish, 31–2
symptoms, 31
types of (See Cluster headache; Migraine;
   Tension-type headache)
head injury
aetiology, 130
associations/risk factors, 130–1
complications, 133–4
   brain abscess, 133
   cranial nerve injury, 133
   CSF leak/meningitis, 133
   dementia pugilistica, 134
   epilepsy, 133
   hydrocephalus, 133
   hypopituitarism, 134
   post-concussion symptoms, 133
conditions related to trauma, 139
defined, 130
differential diagnoses, 134
epidemiology, 130
examination, 131
general approach/management, 130, 132
history, 131
immediate clincal management, 131
investigations, 131
management, 132–3
pathology/pathogenesis, 131
prognosis, 134
secondary brain insults, 132
severity, 134
Heel–shin testing, 20
herniation syndromes, 122–6
5-HT1 agonists, 52, 53
Huntington's disease (HD), 89
defined, 89
history, 89
investigations, 89
management, 89
hydranencephaly, 160
hydrocephalus, 73, 156
aetiology, 155
   communicating, 155
   obstructive, 155
associations/risk factors, 155
complications, 159
   ETV, 159
   shunts, 159
defined, 155
differential diagnoses, 160
epidemiology, 155
examination, 156–7
history, 156
investigations
   CSF drainage tests, 158
   CT head scan, 157
   ICP monitoring, 158
   MRI scan, 157
   neuropsychological testing, 158
   shunt series, 158
medical treatment, 158
pathology/pathogenesis, 155

hydrocephalus (*Continued*)
  prognosis, 159
  surgical treatment, 158–9
  ventricles, CT head scan, 157
hypoglossal nerves, 5
hypopituitarism, 134

ibuprofen, 52
idiopathic intracranial hypertension (IIH),
    32, 54
indapamide, 56, 62
inflammatory myopathies
  aetiology, 115
  associations/risk factors, 115
  complications, 116
  defined, 114
  differential diagnoses, 116
  epidemiology, 115
  examination, 115
  history, 115
  investigations, 115
  management, 116
  pathology/pathogenesis, 115
  prognosis, 116
interstitial oedema, 123
intracerebral haemorrhage, 65, 143
  aetiology, 65
  complications, 67
  defined, 65
  differential diagnoses, 64, 67, 139
  epidemiology, 65
  examination, 65–6
  history, 65
  investigation, 66–7
  management, 67
    non-surgical, 67
    surgical, 67
  non-surgical management, 67
  pathogenesis, 65
  prognosis, 67
  risk factors, 65
  surgical management, 67
intracranial pressure (ICP), raised, 122–6
  aetiology of
    cerebral blood volume, 122
    cerebral oedema, 122–3
    CSF volume, 122
    intracranial mass lesion, 122
  cerebral herniation, 125–6
  complications
    visual loss, 125
  defined, 122
  differential diagnoses, 126
  examination, 124
  history, 123–4
  investigations
    monitoring, 124
    OR signs, 124
  management, 124
    cerebral protection, 125
    reduction, 124
  normal skull growth, prevention of, 123
  pathology/pathogenesis
    Monro–Kellie doctrine, 123
  prognosis, 126

intravenous thrombolysis, 61
ipsilateral hemiplegia, 141

Jefferson's fracture, 148

Lambert–Eaton myasthenic syndrome, 23,
    111–13
  aetiology, 111
  associations/risk factors, 111
  complications, 112
  defined, 111
  differential diagnoses, 113
  epidemiology, 111
  examination, 111–12
  history, 111
  investigations
    blood tests, 112
    intravenous edrophonium test, 112
    neurophysiology, 112
  management, 112
  pathology/pathogenesis, 111
  prognosis, 113
Lambert–Eaton myasthenic syndrome
    (LEMS), 23
Lennox–Gastaut syndrome, 79
Lewy Body dementia, 120
lorazepam, 165
lumbar puncture, 25–7, 32, 39, 54, 70, 91,
    92, 93, 124, 143, 158, 160
Lyme disease, 10, 15, 93

Meniere's disease, 39, 40
meningitis, 31
  aetiology, 91
  complications, 92
  defined, 91
  differential diagnoses, 92–3
  epidemiology, 91
  examinations, 91
  history, 91
  investigations, 91, 92
  management, 92
  pathogenesis, 91
  prognosis, 92
metastatic disease, 151, 152
methysergide, as prophylactic agents for
    headache, 53
MG. *See* Myasthenia gravis (MG)
migraine, 10, 31, 32, 40, 51, 52, 64.
    See also headache
  aetiology, 51
  categories, 51
  epidemiology, 51
  history, 51
    with aura, 51
    without aura, 51
  investigations, 51
  management, 51–2
    prophylactic agents, 52
    prophylactic treatment, 52
MND. *See* motor neurone disease (MND)
mononeuropathies
  aetiology, 104
    median nerve palsy, 104
    peroneal nerve palsy, 104–5

radial nerve palsy, 104
ulnar nerve palsy, 104
defined, 104
diagnosis, 107
epidemiology, 104
history/examination, 105
nerve palsies with symptoms and
signs, 105
Tinel's sign, 105
investigations, 107
management, 107
axon loss, 107
demyelinating conduction block, 107
pathology/pathogenesis, 105
motor neurone disease (MND), 108–10
aetiology, 108
genetic, 108
sporadic, 108
complications, 110
defined, 108
differential diagnoses, 110
epidemiology, 108
examination, 109
history, 108
investigations, 109
management, 109
antispasticity agents, 109
riluzole, as antiglutamate agent, 109
pathology/pathogenesis, 108
PBP, 108
primary lateral sclerosis (PLS), 108
prognosis, 110
progressive bulbar palsy (PBP), 108
progressive muscular atrophy
(PMA), 108
risk factors, 108
motor unit potential (MUP), 22
movement disorders, 88
aetiology, 88
chorea, 89
defined, 88
dystonia, 90
essential (familial) tremor, 88–9
Huntington's disease, 89
hypokinetic, 88
Wilson's disease, 89–90
multiple sclerosis (MS), 7, 39, 80
aetiology, 80
associations/risk factors, 80
complications, 82
defined, 80
differential diagnoses, 82–3
epidemiology, 80
examinations, 81
history, 80–1
investigations, 81–2
management, 82
pathology/pathogenesis, 80
prognosis, 82
rating scale, 81
muscle diseases, 114–17
approach to diagnosis, 114
inflammatory myopathies (*See* inflammatory
myopathies)
inherited muscular dystrophies, 117

muscle, smooth contraction, 23
muscle strength grading, 17
myasthenia gravis (MG), 23, 37, 111–13
aetiology, 111
associations/risk factors, 111
complications, 112
defined, 111
differential diagnoses, 113
epidemiology, 111
examination, 111–12
history, 111
investigations
blood tests, 112
intravenous edrophonium test, 112
neurophysiology, 112
management, 112
immune therapy, 112
medical, symptomatic, 112
thymectomy, 112
pathology/pathogenesis, 111
prognosis, 113
myotonic dystrophy, 117

nerve conduction studies (NCS), 22
axonal disease, 22
conduction velocity, 22
motor element of, 22
myelinated fibres, motor/sensory
functions, 22
nerve palsies, 105. *See also*
mononeuropathies
median, 104
peroneal, 104–5
radial, 104, 106
symptoms and signs, 105
ulnar, 104, 106
neuroanatomy, 4
brainstem, 4–5
cerebellum, 5
cortical anatomy, 4
motor speech area, 4
primary motor cortex, 4
primary visual cortex, 4
Wernicke's area, 4
cortical surface anatomy
cerebral hemisphere, lateral surface, 4
cranial nerves (CN), 4–5
peripheral nervous system, 6
spinal cord, 6
cross section of, 6
vascular anatomy, 5–6
Circle of Willis, 5
neurofibromatosis type 2, 39
neurological examination, 7–9
cranial nerve, 11–16
lesions, signs and symptoms, 12–16
history, 9–11
mental function and speech, 12
power testing, 17
reflex testing, 17
signs and localisation, 7
brief temporal and clues, for particular
aetiological group, 9
suggested order, 11
testing tone, 16–17

neurological examination (*Continued*)
UMN *vs.* LMN lesions, 17
upper/lower limbs, 16
gait assessment, 20
power testing, 17
reflexes, 17–8
sensory, 19–20
tone, 16–17
neurological investigations, 21
electroencephalogram (EEG), 21, 22, 35,
75, 121, 128, 160, 165
electromyography (EMG), 22–3, 110, 112,
113, 116, 117
evoked potential studies, 21–2
nerve conduction studies (NCS), 22, 101, 110
neuroradiology, 23
angiography, 25, 55, 67, 71, 153
computed tomography (CT), 23, 66, 71, 95,
136–8, 140, 142, 149, 150, 157
magnetic resonance imaging (MRI), 23–5,
32, 37, 47, 55, 79, 83, 86, 90, 93, 98,
110, 132, 139, 153, 173, 178, 180, 181
Nocardia, 96
normal pressure hydrocephalus (NPH), 121,
155, 156, 158, 159
numbness, 44
basic investigations, 45
basic management, 45
clinical conditions, 45
defined, 44
selected questions to ask/facts to establish, 44
nystagmus, 11, 13, 40, 78, 81

odontoid peg fracture, 148
oligoclonal bands, 26
optic chiasm, 37

Parkinson's disease, 84
aetiology, 84
complications, 87
differential diagnoses, 86, 87
epidemiology, 84
examinations, 85
history, 84–5
investigations, 85
^{18}F-dopa PET scanning, 86
management, 85–7
dopaminergic therapy, 85
pathology, 84
prognosis, 87
perindopril, as antihypertensive agent, 56, 62
peripheral nerve lesions, 104–7. *See also*
mononeuropathies
peripheral neuropathies' syndromes, 100–3.
See also Guillain-Barré syndrome (GBS)
defined, 100
differential diagnoses, 102
epidemiology, 100
examination, 101
history, 100–1
investigations, 101
extensive blood testing, 101
lumbar puncture, 101
nerve conduction studies (NCS), 101
management, 102

phenytoin, 72, 77, 78, 128, 165
risk factor, 165
polymyositis, 113
posttraumatic amnesia (PTA), 131
propranolol, 52, 89
proptosis, 38, 169
ptosis, 11, 13, 38, 69, 111, 112, 117,
178
pulmonary embolism (PE), 62, 63

radial nerve, 18, 106
palsy, 58, 64, 101, 104, 105
radiculopathy, 41, 43–5, 97
aetiology, 97
associations/riskfactors, 97
complications, 99
cauda equina syndrome (CES), 99
define, 97
examination
cervical spine, 97–8
lumbosacral spine, 97, 98
history, 97
cervical discs, 97
lumbar discs, 97
investigations
cervical spine, 99
lumbosacral spine, 98–9
management
cervical spine, 99
lumbosacral spine, 99
pathology/pathogenesis, 97
Romberg's test, 20, 46, 47

SAH. *See* subarachnoid haemorrhage (SAH)
SCI. *See* spinal cord injury (SCI)
scoliosis, 147
SE. *See* status epilepticus (SE)
seizures, 10, 21, 34, 35, 58, 63, 68, 75, 76,
79, 133, 151, 165, 170, 173. *See also*
epilepsy
febrile seizures of childhood, 79
Lennox–Gestaut syndrome, 76, 79
partial, 75–6
primary generalised, 75
West syndrome, 76, 79
sensory disturbance, 20, 44
basic investigations, 45
basic management, 45
clinical conditions, 45
selected questions to ask/facts to
establish, 44
simvastatin, 56, 62
skull fractures
aetiology, 135
associations/ risk factors, 135
clinical conditions, 139
complications, 138
CT scan, 136–8, 140
defined, 135
differential diagnosis, 143
epidemiology, 135
examination, 136–7
history, 135
investigations, 137–8
management, 138

pathology/pathogenesis, 135
prognosis, 138
sodium valproate, 52, 77–9
somatosensory evoked potentials (SSEP), 21
spasticity, 42, 61, 63, 81, 144
spinal cord
  cross section, 6
  dorsal column, 6
  lateral corticospinal tract, 6
  lateral spinothalamic tract, 6
  lesions, 21
  vascular supply, 6
spinal cord injury (SCI)
  aetiology, 144
  associations/risk factors, 144
  cervical spine fractures, 148
    CT scans, 149–50
  complications, 146
    autonomic dysreflexia, 146
    DVT/PE, 147
    pressure sores, 147
    renal impairment, 147
    respiratory infections, 147
    scoliosis, 147
    spasticity and contractures, 147
    suicide, 147
    syringomyelia, 147
    treatment, 147
    urinary tract sepsis, 147
  cord syndrome, 144
  defined, 144
  differential diagnoses, 148
  epidemiology, 144
  examination, 145
  history, 145
  incomplete spinal cord injury
      syndromes, 144
  investigations, 146
  management, 146
    acute, medical management, 146
  pathology/pathogenesis, 145
    spinal shock, 145
  prognosis, 147
  without radiographic abnormality, 144
spinal extradural metastases (SEM), 41
status epilepticus (SE)
  management of, 79, 165
    airway and breathing, 165
    continuing seizures, 165
    malnourished/alcoholic patients, 165
stenting, 63
steroid therapy, 153
stroke
  complications after, 63
  differential diagnoses, 64
  natural history, 63
  prognosis, 63
  rehabilitation, 63
subarachnoid haemorrhage (SAH), 31, 68,
      134, 143
  aetiology, 68
  cardiovascular signs, 70
  complications, 73–4
  defined, 68
  differential diagnosis, 74

epidemiology, 68
examinations, 69–70
  WFNS grading, 69
history, 68–9
investigations, 70–1
  angiography, 71
  CT cerebral angiogram, 71–2
  CT head, 70
  lumbar puncture, 70
  MRI head, 70–1
management, 71–3
  aneurysm, treatment of, 72
  cerebral vasospasm, prevention and
      treatment, 72–3
meningism, 70
ocular haemorrhage, 70
pathogenesis, 68
prognosis, 74
risk factors, 68
symptoms, 69
WFNS grading, 69–70
subdural empyema, 93, 96
subdural haematoma
  aetiology, 135
  associations/ risk factors, 135
  clinical conditions, 139
  complications, 138
  CT scan, 136–8, 140
  defined, 135
  differential diagnosis, 143
  epidemiology, 135
  examination, 136–7
  history, 135
  investigations, 137–8
  management, 138
  pathology/pathogenesis, 135
  prognosis, 138
sumitriptan, 53
syringomyelia, 147

temperature sensation, 20
tension-type headache
  history, 52
  management, 52
  prophylactic agent, 52
thromboembolic stroke, 59
  aetiology, 59–60
  clinical syndromes, 60
    lacunar stroke, 60–1
    partial anterior circulation stroke, 60
    posterior circulation stroke, 60
    total anterior circulation stroke, 60
  complications, after stroke, 63
  defined, 59
  differential diagnoses, 64
  epidemiology, 59
  history/examination, 60
  investigations, 61
  lacunar stroke (LACS), 60–1
  management, 61–3
    aspirin intake, 61
    carotid endarterectomy, 63
    nutrition and feeding, 62
    rehabilitation, 63
    stenting, 63

thromboembolic stroke (*Continued*)
   stroke units, 61
    thrombolysis, 61
    thromboprophylaxis, 62
    without atrial fibrillation, 62
  partial anterior circulation stroke (PACS), 60
  posterior circulation stroke (POCS), 60
  prognosis, 63–4
  stroke units, role of, 61
  total anterior circulation stroke (TACS), 60
thrombolysis, 61
  medical management, 62
   antiplatelet options, 62
   atrial fibrillation, 62
   cholesterol-lowering treatment, 62
   recombinant tissue plasminogen activator,
    facts related to, 61
TIAs. *See* transient ischaemic attacks (TIAs)
topiramate, 52, 78, 89
Toxoplasmosis, 96
transient ischaemic attacks (TIAs), 55
  ABCD2 score, to estimate risk of stroke,
   57–8
  aetiology, 55
  amaurosis fugax, 55
  aspirin, 56–7
  associations/risk factors, 55
  clinical features, 55
  defined, 55
  differential diagnoses, 58
  epidemiology, 55
  investigations, 55–6
  lifestyle modifications, 57
  management, 55–6
   anticoagulants, 56
   antiplatelet agents, 56
   cholesterol-lowering agents:, 56
   dabigatran, 56
   surgical, 57
  prevention, 55
  prognosis, 57–8
  surgical management, 57
traumatic brain injury (TBI), 130
tremor, 88. *See also* movement disorders;
   stroke
  defined, 88
  essential (familial) tremor, 88–9
trigeminal neuralgia (TN), 54
tumours
  anaplastic astrocytoma, 171
  astrocytic, 169–71
  bone, 144
  brain, 65, 151
  cerebral lymphoma, 176
  cerebral metastases, 151
  craniopharyngioma, 179
  embryonal, 171
  endodermal sinus, 180
  ependymal, 171
  epidermoid/dermoid, 180
  germ cell, 179
  glioblastoma multiforme, 65, 152, 153, 169
  glomus jugulare, 181
  malignant glial, 96

  meningioma, 42, 97, 121, 124, 177
  metastatic, 96, 176
  multicystic, 179
  nasofrontal, 12
  neuroepithelial, 151, 173–4
  neurofibroma, 177–8
  pineal, 172–3
  pituitary adenoma, 151, 153, 178
  schwannoma, 177
  thymic, 112

ulnar nerve, 44, 101, 106
  palsy, 104, 105

vagus nerve, 5, 15, 16
vascular
  abnormality, 65
  aetiology affecting ophthalmic arteries/
   veins, 37
  anatomy (cranial)
   Circle of Willis, 5
  dementia, 118, 120
  injury leading to ischemia or infarct, 6
  lesions, 12, 71
  malformations, 77, 143
  proliferation, 169
venous plexus, 27
verapamil, 53
vertigo, 39
  clinical conditions, 39–40
  defined, 39
  differential diagnoses, 39
  Hallpike manoeuvre, 39–40
  selected questions to ask/facts to
   establish, 39
vestibular neuronitis, 39, 40
visual disturbances, 36–8
  lesion along visual pathway, 36
  local eye disease, 36
  optic nerve disturbance, 36, 37
   persistent visual loss, 37
   transient visual loss, 37
  posterior visual pathways, disturbance
   of, 37
  transient episodic, 37
  visual loss, 36
visual evoked potentials (VEP), 21
visual loss. *See* visual disturbances
VP shunt failure, differential diagnoses of, 160

weakness of legs, 41
  basic investigations, 42
  basic management, 42
  differential diagnoses, 42
  selected questions to ask/facts to
   establish, 41–2
Wernicke's encephalopathy, 121, 127, 128
West syndrome, 22, 79
Wilson's disease, 89–90
  aetiology, 89–90
  defined, 89
  epidemiology, 89
  investigation, 89–90
  management, 89–90